MW01598612

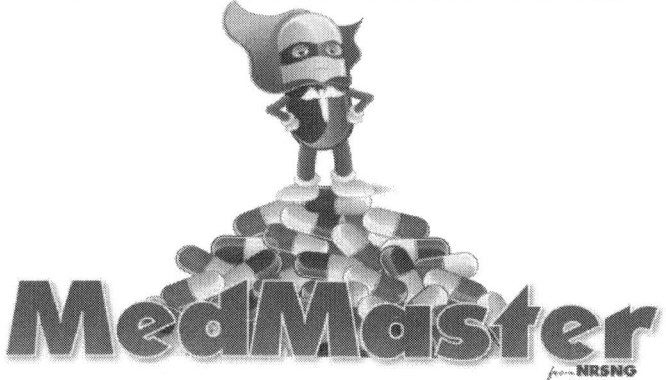

Your Free Gift!

As a way of saying thanks for your purchase, I'm offering a free PDF download:

"63 Must Know NCLEX® Labs"

With these charts you will be able to take the 63 most important labs with you anywhere you go!
You can download the 4 page PDF document by going to NRSNG.com/labs

NCLEX® Essentials
MED SURG

The NCLEX® Doesn't Have to be so DAMN Hard!

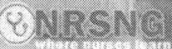

36 NURSING
Cheat Sheets for Students

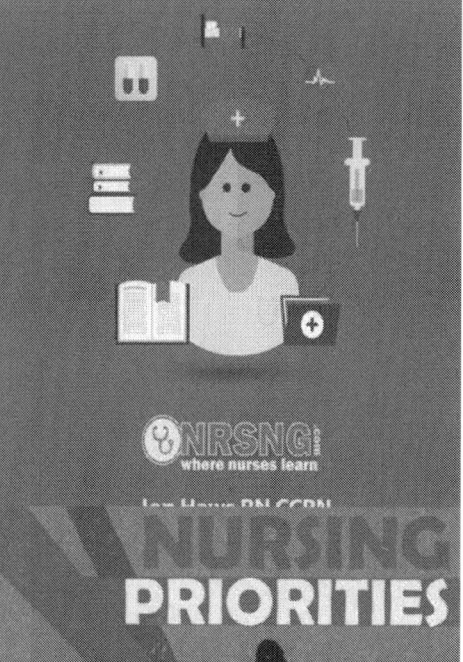

Jen Hays, RN CCRN

Nursing
Case Studies

Pneumothorax
Pancreatitis
Acidosis
CABG
STEMI
Sepsis
DKA
Stroke
Seizures
COPD
ESRD
CHF
More . . .

NURSING
PRIORITIES

5 step approach to making quick decisions in nursing care

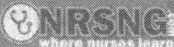

Introduction

Hi! My name is Jon Haws RN BSN CCRN with NRSNG.com. Most of you probably already know me and our company.

If you are new to us . . . it's nice to "meet" you!

Yep . . . unlike some of the other authors and nursing student mentors out there . . . We Are **ACTUALLY** nurses. And pretty damn proud of it too! That's why we are so transparent about who we are, our experiences, and our struggles.

Our goal at NRSNG.com is to **change nursing education**. If you have ever found yourself frustrated with boring lectures, professors that don't seem to care, or incomprehensible PowerPoint's . . . then you've come to the right place.

This book is a combination of some of our most popular books. This is a pretty massive resource at over 42,200 words. **Use the table of contents** to jump between books, sections, chapters etc.

Let me ask you a quick favor. If this book helps you please take a minute to share it with a nursing buddy and leave a quick review on Amazon.com

Check out these Resources from NRSNG.com:

- MedMaster Course: Online Pharmacology Course
  - o (MedMasterCourse.com)
- Med of the Day Podcast: Pharm and Nursing Podcast
  - o (MedoftheDay.com)
- NRSNG Academy: FREE NCLEX® Prep Videos
  - o (NRSNGacademy.com)
- RN Crush!: NCLEX® Prep App
  - o (RNcrush.com)

This is just a small sample of the resources we have created. If you would like to learn more please visit: NRSNG.com and sign up for our FridayFreebie emails.

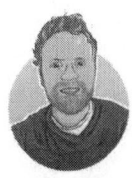

To Your Success!

Jon Haws RN BSN CCRN
Founder and Lead Teacher NRSNG.com

p.s. please take a minute and email me . . . tell me what you *biggest challenge* in nursing school is right now. **contact@nrsng.com.**

Table of Contents

Nursing Priorities
5 Step Approach to Making Quick Decisions in Nursing Care

NRSNG.com | NursingStudentBooks.com
Jon Haws RN CCRN
Sandra Haws RD CNSC

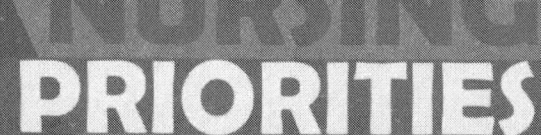

NURSING
PRIORITIES

5 step approach
to making quick decisions
in nursing care

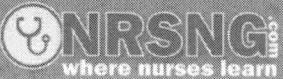

Introduction

It is my privilege to work closely with thousands of nursing students through the blog NRSNG.com and the podcasts NRSNG and Med of the Day. I love it and ask that students reach out to me with their specific questions. I love when students reach out to me to ask specific questions regarding their nursing care and how to improve as a nurse.

After some time I started to kind of aggregate all of the questions coming in and determined that one of the main core concerns for a lot of students and new nurses is how to best prioritize the care, the learning, the school and everything in order able to take care of the patient, in order to grow into the nurse that they – that we all want to be, to grow into a great nurse that can take good care of patients and is a great resource for others and more than anything is able to make an impact in their patients' lives.

After reading through the emails from incredible students and nurses I decided the best thing that I could do was to provide a framework to help prioritize patient care.

I'm going to share with you what I believe are the most important aspects of prioritization. This is by no means a complete list, and it is important to realize that prioritization is the number one most important AND complicated aspect of nursing.

New nurses and experienced nurses alike struggle with this every single shift. This is simply a short framework to help you work through difficult situations while on the floor.

The information contained herein is not new necessarily, but I believe the way it is organized and outlined will be of great benefit to you in your work and school.

Safety

The first topic that we are going to cover is patient safety. Now that may surprise some of you that the first thing is not airway breathing, circulation or something like that and why the first topic that I want to talk about is actually patient safety.

The reason is that patient safety comes into play in every aspect of our nursing care.

Making our patients safe before everything else allows us to take the best care of them, allows us to be prepared and ensures that our patients aren't in any harm and that envelops the ABCs, medication administration, pain . . . really everything else that is involved in nursing care. So for that reason, our primary prioritization focus is patient safety.

When you show for your shift, you get your report. You walk into your patient's room. The very first thing you need to be doing is looking at patient safety.

At the hospital where I work, we have what are called "safety checks". You walk in the room and there are a couple of things you're doing. Whenever I walk into my patient's room, the first thing I'm doing is looking right at the patient and making a quick scan up and down, head to toe, of the patient, their general status, what they look like to me, any visual assessment that I can get very quickly by just glancing at them.

After that, my eyes look up to the monitor. I want to look at what their current vitals are. I want to know what the heart rate is. I want to know what they've been trending. I'm going to compare that with the report I received and what my trends have been for the past day or so.

I look at the patient, scan them up and down, look at the monitor, see what their vitals have been and then I'm going to look at their pump, see what medications they're getting and look at their ventilator and see what their settings are and how well they are supporting the patient.

That will be my quick initial scan for patient safety as I walk into the room. Each of those things plays a specific role in determining how safe my patient is. Basically, I want to look at them and quickly assess that they're not in any sort of visual distress.

Then I'm going to look more closely at that monitor. I'm going to ensure that there isn't any sort of physiologic distress very quickly just based on vital signs. Then I'm going to look closely at the pump and the ventilator and I'm going to make sure that they're not in any sort of mechanical or pharmacologic stress.

As I look at that ventilator, I'm going to make sure the settings are appropriate. I'm going to make sure all their numbers are appropriate and that the patient is receiving the support they need.

As I look at the pump, if they're on any sort of drips, or pressors I'm going to assess that the right medication is programmed in there and that the right concentration and the right rate is all being administered appropriately.

That's my initial first minute of walking into the room.

After that I insure that there are suction canisters available. You never know if you will need these or when you will need these. But I want a suction canister available hooked up with a Yonker so that if something were to go awry, I have that available.

As with most things in life, you never really appreciate how important something is until you need it.

I remember one night in particular I was set to receive a critical patient in the middle of the night. I had my room completely set up and ready for the patient. The hospital that was transferring the patient notified me that they would be flying over on the helicopter to get them to us as fast as possible.

Minutes later I heard the chopping of the helicopter as it landed on the roof of our hospital. Within seconds the two flight nurses came sprinting off the elevator. Racing down the hall toward the room where I was waiting to receive the patient. It is always concerning when Life Flight is running down the hospital hallway. . . this doesn't happen often.

As the go racing down the hall they are yelling "We need suction!". The patient was actively vomiting and increasingly lethargic.

I am forever grateful that I had taken the time to set up the room and prepare suction prior to the patient arriving. I suctioned out her airway and the patient was spared from aspiration.

Though this seems like a minuet detail . . . make sure you have your suction canisters!

After checking for suction canisters I am going to make sure that the bed is in the low position and that my side rails are up, that the bed is locked and more often than not, make sure that the bed alarm is on.

I'm going to make sure there's enough light in the room for the patient to see and I'm going to make sure that I have an Ambu bag, that I have any sort of resuscitative equipment that I'm going to need for my patient.

Murphey's Law states: "What Can Go Wrong Will Go Wrong"

This may seem pessimistic but in nursing a better way to think of it is simply being prepared for any situation that might occur in your patients room. Our ultimate goal is to give our BEST to each and every patient. That includes simply being prepared for the worst.

The smart nurse, the smart student is going to accept that things go bad. Things can go bad and things will go bad.

So the smart student and the smart nurse are going to accept that. Things can and will go wrong. Hopefully, you don't learn this lesson from something going wrong due to lack of preparedness.

Being prepared includes things like an Ambu bag and suction canisters. That's going to include that your patient has IV access. You cannot anticipate every variable, but having the basics prepared is essential to nursing.

The next thing I'm going to look at is restraints. I know in nursing school they teach to never use restraints. Never, ever, ever use restraints.

So when I came out of nursing school, I kind of adopted the mindset that restraints were in and of themselves a bad thing. Well, here's my take on it now.

Restraints aren't something that we just put on every patient. They're not something that we do just so that we can make our night easier, make our day easier. They're not something we do just because a patient has ticked us off or anything like that. That's not the reason for restraints.

The reason for restraints is to protect the patient . . . to keep them safe.

It's to protect the patient from interfering with the care that they need in order to actually get better. It's not so that they don't hit us. It's not so that we can just keep them in bed. They are a tool to help the patient get the care that they need in order to improve, in order to be safe.

Now again, like I said, I was always kind of leery of restraints just based on teachings in nursing school. However, when I really learned my lesson was after I had my first patient extubate themselves.

This was just a terrible experience for me because I always want my patients to safe and comfortable. I want them to get better. But in this case I also granted far too much leeway to these patients who were confused, were combative, and who needed to be ventilated.

As they were being ventilated, to ensure that they were able to keep their tube in and seeing that they were aggressive and going for the tube, it was important to restrain them.

I allowed the restraints to be tied not as tight as they should have been and allowed the patient to move around in bed and get to the point that he was able to pull that tube out. Someone ran in the room and saw this and yelled my name. I immediately knew what had happened. I ran into the room and fortunately the patient was okay, we were able to bag them for a little bit, put them on a Ventimask and then transferred them very quickly to a nasal cannula.

This experience helped me to learn that restraints are a safety tool. It's for the patient to be OK and to be safe. That is why we use them.

I believe safety is number one. It's number one. It's everything that we do as a nurse and it is truly how we help heal individuals.

In fact in a 2000 article from the Institute of Medicine, entitled _To Err is Human: Building a Safer Healthcare System_, they bring to light how many errors occur in hospitals to the point of causing patient death.

They discovered in this article is that as many as 98,000 people die in the hospital each year as a result of preventable medical errors.

I know that's not talking specifically to safety necessarily but as we make safety our number one goal, our number one priority, we're going to prevent these medical errors.

Ninety-eight thousand patients die due to professionals, medical professionals lapsing on patient safety or allowing these preventable medical errors to occur.

That's a huge number and that is why I truly, truly believed safety is the number one priority. That's everything that you need to be focusing on.

Now in order to be a safe nurse, I believe there are three qualities that the nurse must possess.

Number one is knowledge.
Number two is a backbone.
Number three is they actually have to give a crap. They actually have to care.

So why do I think these three things are the most important?

Well, first of all, knowledge. Knowledge. If you don't understand what can go wrong, you're not going to be able to keep your patient from those things going wrong.

Being a nurse isn't the same as working in a corporate office where you can put a decimal in the wrong place and the company loses money (which I did in a previous life . . . story for another time).

Being a nurse is different than working in fast food where being late on an order makes a patient upset.

Working as a nurse, we truly have patients' lives in our hands. What that requires of us is that we learn everything we can.

You're learning the procedures. You're learning how to start IVs. But beyond learning how to start IVs, you're learning why we start IVs, why we do them a certain way, why we assess for induration and redness and swelling. You're learning those things – and all the appendages around the procedures are to keep our patients safe.

So learning how to chart on whatever system you're using, learning how to scan the meds, learning how to scan the badge, learning what boxes to check, those are all good and important. But learning why we do those things, learning what can go wrong if we don't do those things right, are so much more important. That's why I believe knowledge is very important to keep our patients safe.

Number two is a backbone. By having a backbone, I mean that you are willing to advocate for your patients. Now I know patient advocacy and everything is something that's talked about a lot in nursing school. You may not realize why until you're actually out working. But being an advocate for your patient requires that you question things, that you're not accepting everything as truth with orders and with order sets and things, that you're thinking through things, that you're having a backbone to say, "I'm not sure I understand why we're doing this."

People make mistakes. Doctors are busy. They may not even truly know the full patient history. You're the nurse. You're there. You have a role in ensuring that your patient is safe. Part of having a backbone is being willing to admit when you're not sure, admit when you have a question.

I was always afraid going into nursing that I would get my job on a floor where there was a tremendous amount of cattiness and backbiting and older nurses hating the young.

But I don't think that's the case nowadays or at least that hasn't been my experience. I think all those horror stories are a lot like these teenage high school movies. It's more just to create drama in the field. I don't think that older nurses or the more experienced nurses are out there to get you. There may be some like that. But that hasn't been my experience.

From my experience, older nurses want to help you succeed because they want to work with nurses who care, who try their best. So having a backbone includes being willing and being in tune enough to recognize when you're not sure how to do something and then going and asking to get the help that you need.

Number three, you have to give a crap. Now this is an obvious one. In order to keep your patients safe, you have to actually care that they're going to be safe. That's kind of obvious but I think it's important as well, because you do see nurses that just don't seem to care. But doing these safety checks, keeping your patients safe, it makes everything go much easier.

Families will respect you more. It makes the patient respect you and insures that the patient is safe. In the end, you can't prevent every possible scenario. Things will go wrong. Patients will get hurt. Patients will pass away on your watch. But you can care and you can try and you can do your best when you're at the job and when you're working with those patients.

So again, patient safety and keeping your patients safe needs to be your number one priority with your nursing care. So when it comes down to how to prioritize your care, I think if you're looking at keeping your patients safe, that's going to be the number one thing.

Use some of the strategies I've suggested here, do your own research and read.

I believe that keeping your patients safe comes number one as it entails and envelops everything else in our nursing care.

So just take a deep breath. Relax and as you're putting your patient safe, everything will come in line. Don't overstress yourself part of keeping your patients safe includes making sure that you're not getting in over your head. Don't be afraid to say, "I don't know that I'm capable of this. I'm not sure that I'm comfortable with this."

Just take a step back. Relax. Learn everything you can and realize that this is a hard job. This is a hard career. It's physically. It's emotionally, spiritually. It's just draining. It's just a draining job.

But as you're trying to keep your patients safe, you will find that other things will start to come in line.

So I believe safety is the number one thing you need to be focusing on is your patient safe. And the very close second is going to be airway, breathing and circulation. I think it ties in very directly to safety. The two kind of go hand in hand.

As you're assessing safety, you're kind of also assessing airway, breathing and circulation.

So why airway, breathing and circulation? Those are the ABCs, right? We talk about that all the time. Now, as you know, the BLS guidelines have changed from ABCs to CAB. So of course if you're in a situation where you're providing BLS, you need to focus CAB, circulation, airway and breathing. Of course the reason for doing that is because by pumping the heart, you're getting oxygen moving throughout the body.

In an assessment situation, you're going in and dealing with your patients and as you're prioritizing your care, you need to focus airway, breathing, circulation.

The reason for that of course is pretty obvious. You want your patients to be breathing. You want to make sure they have a clear patent airway in order to breathe and that they're actually perfusing.

So how can you check for airway, breathing and circulation?

First of all is airway. The first thing you want to do with your patient is you want to assess their level of consciousness. Are they awake and alert enough to maintain their airway? Is their neurological status stable or is it beginning to decline?

Now if your neurological status is beginning to decline, of course there's going to concern you that the airway is going to become compromised. That needs to be at the forefront of your mind. Again that plays directly in with safety.

But you definitely need to be very closely monitoring their consciousness and to see if their ability to maintain the airway is continued.

As you're assessing the level of consciousness you need to think, " What's going to be the reasons that my patient may be declining neurologically? Is it some sort of neuro trauma or is possibly due to blood sugars? Could it be due to the blood gas? Is the reason that their neurological status declining because they are having respiratory problems?"

You are probably are BLS-certified. But with ACLS, there are things that we think about with patient resuscitation called the Hs and Ts.

Now some of these Hs and Ts are going to play in very closely with the patient's ability to maintain their airway.

H's include:
Hypovolemia, Hypoxia, Hydrogen ion (acidosis), Hyper-/hypokalemia, Hypoglycemia, Hypothermia.

T's include:

Toxins, Tamponade(cardiac),Tension pneumothorax, Thrombosis (coronary and pulmonary), Trauma

Walking in on your patient, assessing their airway, you're going to assess that level of consciousness and kind of determine, "Are they going to be able to maintain the airway going forward?"

You're going to want to assess the patient's ability to deep breathe, assess their cough and gag reflex. Even if they're awake but they don't have any sort of cough and gag reflex, they're not going to be able to maintain their secretions. So that's going to definitely be a concern for you.

Then you just want to make sure the airway is clear. Is there anything in their mouth? That might sound kind of ridiculous. But again, as a lot of you know, I work on a neuro ICU and so a lot of our patients are traumatic strokes.

What can oftentimes happen with these patients is of course pocketing food as they aren't able to feel one side of their body. If they're on a regular diet or if they're on a diet, they may be able to pocket food on one side of their mouth.

Recently, I was with a patient who when asked to swallow some pills we noticed in the side of his mouth, there appeared to be something. Very quickly, we had him open his mouth more fully and we found there was an enormous piece of cantaloupe in his mouth from his dinner during the previous shift several hours ago.

Now the patient eventually ended up being placed on BiPAP throughout the night making it a bit scary to think that had we not noticed that huge piece of cantaloupe in there, then throwing him on the BiPAP machine and possibly forcing that cantaloupe into his airway, how terrifying that may have been.

So you are going to want to assess that their airway is clear.

With breathing, of course if our patient is talking, then they're moving air.

But what you're going to want to do is to assess lung sounds, assess how well air is moving between the two lungs. Is the airway moving equally? Is air moving equally between the two lungs? Can we hear air moving? Is one side maybe less than the other? Are they having to work to breathe?

Something that I've noticed with new nurses is that they may just not quite notice if a patient is working to breathe. If the patient is talking, great, their fine they will think – but if you notice that your patient is working to breathe, that's never a good thing.

We know what our respiratory rate should be. So if you assess that your patient is breathing at 45 breaths per minute, why are they doing that? Why are they having to breathe that fast? Are they trying to blow off a tremendous amount of CO_2? What would possibly be the reason for them having all that CO_2?

So if you see a patient breathing that fast, what's the reason for that? Is it anxiety? Is it possibly CO_2? Is there something else going on that's causing the patient to breathe that fast?

If you notice that a patient is becoming possibly more somnolent or that they're breathing very fast, it's never a bad idea to kind of just question the physician and see if you can get an ABG. ABGs are easy to do. They're inexpensive and they're very quick.

So assessing where your patient's PO_2, SaO_2, pCO_2 are is a good way to be able to tell how well-ventilated the patient actually is.

It becomes very easy for us to rely on our pulse oximetry. Now pulse oximetry, obviously I use it and obviously I assess it and determine basic respiratory status based on that. However pulse oximetry can be a very misleading number.

Let's think about what pulse oximetry is measuring. What it's measuring is the percent of oxygenated hemoglobin in the peripheral vascular bed.

So what it's really measuring is how much of our hemoglobin is oxygenated in our peripheral vascular bed. It's not telling us the actual oxygenation of our tissues. So it can be very misleading.

It doesn't matter necessarily how much oxygenated hemoglobin we have in our vascular system if it's not being transported into our tissues. If our tissues are not receiving oxygen, then circulation is basically for naught. That's the whole point of circulation is to oxygenate our peripheral tissues. SpO_2 can't tell us anything about the oxygenation of tissues.

That's why when you have a patient who is ventilated there are blood gases for a reason. We have them hooked up to SpO_2 but we're drawing the blood gasses to tell us a better picture of their actual oxygenation. Beyond that, if you have a patient who's septic, we're drawing SvO_2 to determine oxygen extraction from the blood stream.

Now I know that's a little higher level than we need to get into for this but what I'm trying to tell you is don't just look at the monitor, see your SpO_2 as 96% and assume that everything is fine. That is not the end-all, be-all of airway and breathing determinations. Don't just trust your SpO_2.

You are the nurse. Those are machines and SpO_2 isn't necessarily the best indicator of how well your patient is actually breathing.

Am I beating a dead horse?
So that's airway and breathing. Lastly, we will talk about circulation. What does circulation obviously deal with? Well, that deals with how our blood is moving throughout our body and our volume status.

Firstly, we're going to examine for any signs of bleeding. We're going to examine for perfusion. What's their level of consciousness? Why do we say level of consciousness? Well, we have our blood pressure and then we have our MAP, of course our mean arterial pressure.

What that mean arterial pressure is doing is telling us basically the pressure required to perfuse tissues. We need that number to be above 60. Then we also have our CPP (cerebral perfussion pressure), or the blood pressure required to perfuse the brain tissue. CPP can be a hard number to get because in order to get CPP, we need to get ICP (intracranial pressure).

To get your CPP, you're going to take your MAP and subtract ICP. So ICP is the amount of pressure within your head of course and that's going to range 5 to 15 or so in a normal patient, a patient without any sort of intracranial process.

MAPs, of course must be above 60 as an absolute minimum. Generally, a normal MAP will be 70 or so to 100.

Knowing that we can determine that cerebral perfusion pressure should be between about 70 and 85 (MAP-ICP).

Basically, ICP is the force the MAP must work against to get blood into the brain and is represented as CPP.

As that ICP increases, if MAP doesn't increase along with it, cerebral perfusion pressure is going to decrease perfussion to the brain will be lost.

That is the reason that with circulation, we're going to assess for level of consciousness. They may not be perfusing the brain tissue and that's obviously a very terrifying thing. It can lead to anoxic brain injuries.

We're also going to assess skin color. Check for cyanosis and check pulse rate and blood pressure. Now with pulse rate and blood pressure, of course there's so much more that we can talk about with this, but the two in a lot of situations kind of go hand in hand. If our blood pressure drops, our heart rate will go up to try to maintain that cardiac output (in a healthy individual).

You need to know your patient trends. **Always, always, always** know what your patient is trending. If you have a patient whos blood pressure normally runs 90 over 50 and their MAP is appropriate, then you don't need to worry about their blood pressure rising if that's their normal trend.

However, if you have a patient who's normally trending in 150 over 90 and all of a sudden their blood pressure is down in the 90s over 50s, that's a concern.

So vice versa with that too, blood pressure and pulse are responding to conditions within the body. So it's very important that we assess why the changes are happening in our patient.

ABCs and safety go hand in hand quite closely. But when it comes down to prioritizing your care with your patients, really you have to simultaneously kind of be assessing for safety and for the ABCs.

My advice to you as always is that there are a lot of important things in nursing. There are a lot of required things in nursing and there's more and more being required of us as far as charting and checklists and rounding and things like that, that can detract from your time. But what you need to do is focus on prioritizing patients first.

This is something that I tell to students and new nurses as I precept them is that I never want them to become **checklist nurses**. It's so easy to come to work and we know what we have to do before we can go home. We have to chart this. We have to chart our vitals. We have to chart these things. We have to do all these things before we can go home.

However, a concern for me with new nurses is when they focus entirely on those checklists, those things that have to be done before we go. Those are important things and they need to be done. However, what always comes first is the patient and their well-being. And understanding how these things all play into that.

The checklists and the rounding and charting that we are required to do are kind of failsafe for the hospital. They're to make sure that bad nurses are doing what they should be doing.

But as a good nurse, what you will be doing is you will be doing these things because you want to understand what's going on with the patient and that they're OK and that there are no new concerns.

So always safety and ABCs. Those are the first two things that you need to be prioritizing in your patient care.

We recently had a patient on our floor with a newer nurse taking care of her whos neuro status was declining very rapidly. It was night shift and he was a new nurse and he was concerned about giving her a couple of medications. So he wanted to get a tube, an OG or an NG tube to be able to give the patient her medications.

Now with a patient who isn't opening her mouth and isn't breathing very well, anyway, my initial thought with him was you're probably looking at needing to intubate this patient in order to maintain the airway because the second you insert an NG tube in a patient who's only moderately breathing through the nose your closing off one of their passageways to get air, and sure enough, 30 minutes later, the patient ended up intubated.

With her not breathing through the mouth, she obviously isn't going to be getting air that way. She only has her two nasal passageways to breathe and if one is occluded, you're stuck with one way for this patient to get air.

So that's kind of all the things that you have to think about. What I told him is, "Look, I can't tell you what to do. What I can tell you is kind of the framework to think through this and as the nurse, you need to think through it and make a firm decision and then stick with it."

The best decision in that case will ultimately come down to how well is that patient going to breathe and maintain their airway. Is the patient safe? Are they able to breathe? In the book, the ICU Book, the best critical intensive care book that I have found, Dr. Marino ultimately concludes that it is always appropriate to intubate if you feel that the patient needs to be intubated. There's a lot of different thought processes and checklists for when you should intubate, but ultimately it comes down to, "Do you think the patient needs to be intubated?"

As a nurse, you play a role in that. You really play a very vital role in that. As you're at the bedside assessing the patient, you need to be on the phone with your physician saying, "I do not feel comfortable with this patient. We need to get an airway," and there's a lot of things that you can do to help and to ensure that the patient is safe and is getting the air and the circulation that they need.

Pain

It might seem kind of weird that I'm prioritizing pain as the third thing to focus on. But if we think about it, pain is one of the things that is really hard for us to gauge in our patients.

In nursing school we talked about how pain is the fifth vital sign. The reason for that is because it is something that we cannot quantify ourselves. We can't look at a monitor and see what someone's pain is. We can look at a patient. We can try to assess it but it becomes very hard as your patients become non-verbal or they're unable to really express pain appropriately.

The hard thing too is that everybody interprets and fills and responds to pain differently, between cultures, gender, and between children and adults everyone responds differently to pain. Again, especially as patients become non-verbal, it becomes hard for us to be able to assess the pain.

Now the reason that I prioritize pain below ABCs is because as we know, a lot of the interventions that we have for pain medically are going to be opioids and opioids agonists. So what these things actually do is cause a general CNS depression and by doing that, it can alter the way that we perceive and respond to pain. So it has that positive impact there on how we actually respond to pain.

However, unfortunately by depressing the CNS, it also will play the negative role of lowering heart rate, blood pressure, and respirations. For that reason I placed pain below ABCs and safety. Now let's go into that a little bit deeper.

So if we have a patient who comes in, and their blood pressure is incredibly low, their MAPs are hovering right at 60, maybe just a tad below, their respirations are very low, they're having a hard time getting air, and their pulse is 40, it wouldn't be wise to give three milligrams of morphine or some Dilaudid.

If we decreased the respiratory drive to the point that they're not breathing or if we decrease the heart rate to the point – they go into like an atrioventricular rhythm or symptomatic bradycardia or something, then we've created a problem far beyond the patient experiencing pain.

We recently had a patient come on a recent shift with blood pressures in the 60s over 40s and was experiencing afib with RVR and in an incredible amount of pain due to a recent femur fracture. The risk that we ran with giving her pain medication was that she was highly unstable hemodynamically.

So that was the first and most important thing (ABCs, Safety). Of course we feel terrible for the patient that they're in that pain but we can't treat that pain and cause a bigger problem that could potentially lead to death (hemodynamic instability).

Pain is uncomfortable. Pain is hard for the patient. It's hard for us to see our patients in pain but they aren't going to die from pain.

Therefore pain comes below ABCs. So in the same sense, if we think about patient safety is our number one goal, giving them pain medication when they're hemodynamically unstable compromises the patient's safety.

Now there are other things that we can do. We can do ice packs. We can do compression, elevation, heat packs, things like that, to try to relieve pain, possibly a Tylenol or something like that. But we can't be doing things that are going to compromise the patient's safety and ABCs.

At the same time, one of the most annoying things to patients and to family members is for them to hit the call light, say they're in pain and then to see their nurse chatting it up or laughing or walking around or eating a snack.

If a patient is in pain and they can receive pain medication, that becomes a priority for you, a very urgent priority for you. These patients deserve to be treated and addressed quickly when they're in pain.

When a patient is in the hospital, their priorities become your priorities. I think that's the best way that I could think to express that is that their priorities, their needs become your priorities.

You're no longer on your schedule. I'm no longer on Jon's schedule when I clock in an accept an assignment. I'm doing everything I can to ensure that my patients are safe and well taken care of when I'm on shift and when I'm taking care of them.

Pain is a very real sensation that our patients have and we need to treat it as such. We need to treat it quickly. If they're in pain, we don't say, "OK, well, let me finish this charting real quick and I will be in there in a second." What we do is we go in there and we assess the pain. We determine where it's coming from, why they're having it, what type of pain it is.

We educate our patients on the pain. One of the best things that always works really well is to tell your patient what their pain medications are, what they do and when they're allowed to have them and why we're not just going to give them pain medication at any moment and kind of educate them that they need to call us when they're in pain, if they're capable of doing so, that we're not just going to sneak in the room in the middle of the night and inject some Dilaudid into their IV. But they're actually going to have to be awake and experiencing the pain so that we can assess that and determine the reason for it.

If possible write their pain medications and schedules on the white board in their room.

Every time you give pain medication, it really is important to assess it. You need to assess if it's new, if it's a different kind of pain, especially. I work on that neuro ICU so I'm always checking for neuropathic type pain. Are we having neuropathic type pain? Are we having surgical pain or are we having a new type of pain that maybe would bring up different concerns.

That's going to vary somewhat depending on the type of floor that you work on. So if you're working on a surgical floor, orthopedic floor, the reasons that your patients might experience new pains maybe be different than if you were to work on a med/surg floor or in an ICU.

So that's really kind of the basics of pain. I truly believe pain is very important. If four patient, three of them are stable. They all want medications. They all have medications due. One patient has Protonix due and you're in that room and you're getting prepared. You're thinking of giving that patient their Protonix. Then another patient calls and says they're in excruciating pain.

What becomes the priority? Protonix or the pain? Well, the pain becomes the priority. You never know how long you're going to be stuck in the other patient's room, giving them that Protonix. Protonix isn't urgent. We're not going to save someone's life by giving Protonix right now and we're not going to affect patient satisfaction or anything like that, by giving Protonix right now.

However, going into that room and giving that Protonix and suddenly the patient wants to talk and then they need water and they need ice. All of a sudden, you've delayed giving the pain medication 30 minutes.

If you have a patient who wants pain medication, but you have another patient who needs to be intubated, of course intubation is the priority.

You have two patients next to each other. One just got out of the restraint and they're intubated and they're reaching for their tube. But you're on your way to another patient's room to give them morphine. What becomes the priority? The airway, the safety. You got to take care of the patient who's about to pull their tube out and compromise their airway over getting that pain medication.

If you have a patient who needs pain medication but their pressures are not stable enough to get it, pressures become the priority.

So I hope this is all starting to kind of come together. I hope that you're starting to kind of make sense of everything and kind of what you would really focus on.

And that's why we work with other nurses. That's why we have techs. There are things that we can have other nurses do for us. You can say, "Hey, I need to take care of this patient here. Can someone address the pain situation on my other patient's room?" So that's how you can take care of more than one thing at once. You need to develop good, strong relationships with the nurses you work with, so that you can always have someone to rely on if you become incapable of addressing two priorities at once.

So that's kind of where pain comes in and why pain would be after safety and ABCs. At the same time pain comes so high on the list of priorities because it is incredibly important and the last thing you want to do is to have patients need pain medication or have serious pain and you're lollygagging through the halls and messing around.

Know Your Limitations

Knowing your limitations includes knowing what you understand, knowing what you don't understand and being humble enough and confident enough to understand when you don't understand something and when you need the help of other nurses and other staff and when you should be reaching out for that help.

I know this kind of sounds strange but this truly is part of the prioritization framework because if you do not understand what you know and if you do not understand when you need the help of others, it becomes very dangerous for you to be working with patients. It also becomes very hard for you to correctly think through problems that may arise and this can really lead to dangerous situations for your patients.

There's an excellent article written by Mary Gillespie and Barbara Paterson and it's titled _Helping Novice Nurses Make Effective Clinical Decisions: The Situated Clinical Decision-Making Framework_[1]. There are a couple of things that I really like about this article.

I want to go over a couple of quotes from the article. The first quote is this: _"Novice nurses, new graduates or nurses with limited experience in the care setting in which they work tend to view decision making as responding to patient complaints and following protocols or documented care plans. As they make decisions, their focus leans toward doing rather than on thinking and reflecting. Novice nurses often do not recognize or appreciate the relevance of deviations from the textbook picture of clinical situation."_

So their concern is that because of this it becomes really hard to think through a complete picture. It becomes really hard to see the whole picture. When we can't see the whole picture, it becomes hard for us to correctly respond to deviations, to changes in our patient.

That comes with experience. That comes with seeing things. That comes with working with a varying patient population. So it's hard to say that you just need to develop that skill.

At the same time, that comes with knowledge. That comes with seeking out opportunities to learn and to grow. The authors concern is that as the aging nursing population begins to retire and as more new nurses come in to the field, there's a bigger population of nurses who haven't had that broad spectrum of clinical experience. The other concern is that patients are becoming more sick and you notice if you've been in a hospital, people are becoming sicker and sicker. The complexity of diseases begins to grow and so as a whole, a lot of nurses haven't seen some of the situations they're confronted with.

As we come out of nursing school, we're trained to think from the textbook picture of a patient. But the problem is no patient has just thyroid disease or no patient has just stroke and not every patient is the same. Not every body is the same and the way that people respond to diseases is very different.

So the concern is being able to see the whole picture and being able to understand when you're out of your ability to appropriately respond. What is most important to do is that you get confronted with these more difficult patients and that you have a support system within where you work that you can rely on, other nurses to help you and to teach you through these times.

The best thing you can do while you're an intern or while you're starting a new job, is to seek out the opportunity to work with the most complex patients that you can find while you have that support system, that mentor and that preceptor there with you.

What that does is that gives you that comfort and that safety net as you're working through these complex patients. Then when you get out on your own, you need to build that network of nurses that you can trust and that you can rely on and that are willing to help you.

At the same time, you need to be sure to not just be checking off boxes. Check, check, check. Charting is done. Time to go home. You need to be thinking through the whole picture.

The other quote is, *"When confronted with complex or unfamiliar clinical situations, novice nurses frequently respond by drawing on theoretical knowledge and psychomotor skills rather than enacting decision making that addresses the complex and multidimensional nature of the situation."*

So again kind of like we said, there's not one response necessarily to every patient and it can be hard as a new nurse to see that and to grasp – you can't just do "one thing fixes all" in every patient. Patients respond differently and understanding that is very important.

Knowing your limitations, knowing when you're beyond your limitations and seeking the opportunities to grow and to learn as you become more experienced, that will help you take better care of your patients and prioritize your workload and time.

In the above article they talk about decisions that we're confronted with when things happen in our patients. So some of the decisions that we have to be able to make are, *"Should I wait and watch? Should I try something? Should I inform someone? Should I involve or consult someone else? How do I know if I made the best decision?"*

So when it comes down to priorities, those are kind of the decisions that we have to make when things change with our patients. I think it's really, really hard to see that whole picture every time. So you need to be able to think through that and having that experience really allows you to think through that a little bit better.

I just want to express how important it is to understand your limitations first of all. A lot of times we see nurses that don't reach out and ask questions for whatever reason. To me that's really the most frustrating thing with newer nurses . . . those that don't reach out. With experienced nurses too, it's hard when they don't reach out.

The first thing that I tell every student and every nurse is to ask questions. Ask as many questions as you can think of, that allows those that you work with, the charge nurse, the physicians and the other people that you work with, to understand what your thought process is and knowing that thought process allows them to mentor and to guide you and allows them to trust you. Eventually you're going to be back on the very back end of the unit all by yourself, isolated in the middle of the night, with three patients, four patients, and people need to be able to trust your thought processes and where you're thinking. That comes with time.

But what you can do now is to build a network of people that you can rely on, build the confidence to ask questions and to build the humility to know that people aren't going to judge you for not knowing something. If you haven't been exposed to a situation before, you can't know what to do. It's okay not to know, where the danger happens is when you don't seek the help.

So with any situation, with any prioritization framework, always know your limitations and be willing to express concerns when they arise.

You can do this. Nursing is very hard. Understanding what the best decision to make at any given time is always hard.

You can do this. I would highly suggest that you go and read the article *Helping Novice Nurses Make Effective Clinical Decisions* by Mary Gillespie and Barbara Paterson. Very helpful article, very insightful and it will help you with your decision making framework.

Education

Patient education becomes part of what you're doing the whole time you're working with your families and the patients.

As you're talking with families, as the family's in the room and the patient is starting to crump and you're about to intubate, you can be telling the family basically what you're doing.

"They're having a harder time breathing. In order to help them breathe, we're going to put this tube in their throat and this machine is going to help them breathe."

Just very simple, basic education can go a long way with family members.

In an article from Boston University, they state that at least 20 percent of all patients who are admitted to the hospital make a repeat visit within 30 days of discharge.

It also states in the same article that Medicare alone currently spends 15 billion a year on re-hospitalization. It is very costly to have patients readmitted to the hospital. Educating patients, they found in this article can greatly reduce the amount of readmissions.

It is really hard to pinpoint exactly why these patients are coming back. We can't necessarily say that they were never educated. But it is very clear that – clear discharge instructions as well as educating patients while they're in the hospital can reduce the chance of readmission.

In this study, they found that patients who received clear instructions on what they were receiving, why things were being done, were 30 percent less likely to be readmitted. So it's very important to educate our patients from that standpoint.

Now from another standpoint, what I have found is that educating the family members can greatly improve your relationship with them, which makes the entire stay easier for everyone.

Educating family members and patients I have found creates a much better relationship with them. By improving the relationship with family members and patients, you're then able to take care of them and provide the care that they need in a much less controversial way.

On my floor we admit a lot of stroke patients. They will come in with stroke-like symptoms to the ED. They will be admitted to our floor and of course the patient is NPO. Now family members just hate that. They hate it. They don't understand it. They get very upset about it. The family member hasn't eaten in four hours and they just need to eat or they're going to die, right?

Now, taking a minute to explain to them why they shouldn't be eating can greatly improve the situation. At times you really have to be very straightforward with them saying, "We cannot give food to your family member and have the risk of them choking or the food going down into their airway would compromise their ability to breathe and could potentially lead to death."

Educating patients and if need be, educating them very straightforwardly can help them to understand why we're doing things. I actually recently had a patient who – when I came on the shift, I was told that they had a left side mastectomy. Sure enough I go in there and the patient didn't have a restricted extremity armband on and they actually had an IV in their left arm. They've been taking blood pressures on that side and everything.

I went and I educated the daughter and the patient. The daughter was actually very forceful about the way things were done with her mom, the daughter of the patient. I explained to them why extremities become restricted once they have had a mastectomy on that side.

I educated them on the purpose and they said, "Well, no one has ever told us that before. We didn't know that. No one said anything." I said, "Well, look, I'm sorry that that hadn't been explained before but this is the risk with it and this is kind of what needs to happen." Well, they declined having another IV started but I educated them and said this – "I need to make sure you understand the risks and I need to make sure that you can understand what can happen with lymphedema if that IV continues to be in that side".

I educated them that going forward, they really need to bring that up as she's admitted, they need to say they have the left sided mastectomy and then they need to be sure that professionals, healthcare professionals are not drawing blood or doing IVs on that side.

Just doing that little bit of education will help them not only now but in the future as they go forward in their healthcare. So it really helps. I found that taking that extra minute can save HOURS of time in the end. Of course make sure the patient is safe. Make sure the ABCs are good. Make sure their pain is controlled and make sure that it's a situation that you can handle.

Then what I do is I go in there and I say, "OK, my name is Jon. I'm going to be taking care of you this evening. Here's kind of the plan for this evening. We have these medications that we're going to be giving. These are your pain medications. This is when you can have them. I'm going to be coming in here every two hours to turn. I'm going to be coming in here every hour to check the vitals and earlier in the morning, I'm going to come in to do labs. That's going to be at about 4 o'clock in the morning and then we do have a CT scan. So at about 3:30, 4 o'clock, we're going to go down for the CT scan. That will take a few minutes and then we will come back up here to the room."

Just by providing that little bit of education, you're able to help them. The family and the patients aren't going to be surprised when you come in to do things, because they were made aware previously and you're getting a good understanding that they understand what's going to be happening.

Patient education as far as plan of care, medications and discharge instructions can really go a long way. Taking that time out of your "schedule", that couple of minutes I have found can go just a tremendously long way in keeping the patients happy and satisfied and keeping them on your side and making them feel that you're on their side and you're looking out for their best interest.

Putting it All Together and Decision Fatigue

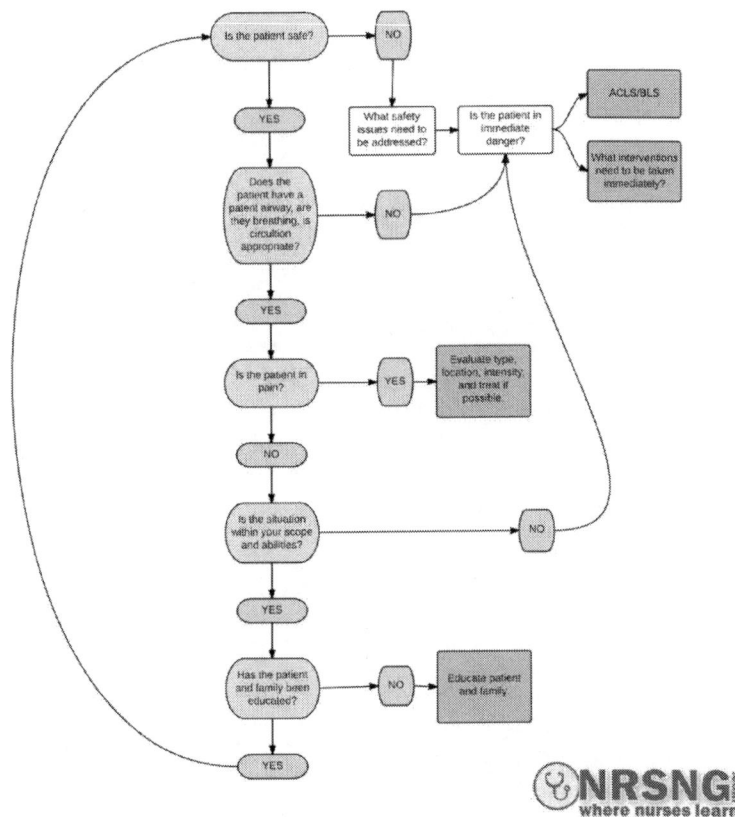

View this chart in full resolution at NRSNG.com/Prioritization

Putting it Together
- Is the patient safe?
- Does the patient have a patent airway, are the breathing, is circulation appropriate?
- Is the patient in pain?
- Is the situation within your scope and abilities?
- Have the patient and/or family been educated?

As you can see from the above chart (you can download a full resolution image at NRSNG.com/Prioritization) prioritization is not a one and done task for the nurse.

Prioritizing our care is highly cyclical and requires that in each and every interaction with the patient we are thinking through this framework. Just because you are able to work fully through the framework during your initial assessment upon starting your shift does not indicate that everything will continue perfectly smooth the rest of the night (obviously).
Do not be hard on yourself if it takes you time to learn prioritization. Even experienced nurses struggle at times with knowing exactly what to do in a given circumstance. As you become more experienced as a nurse the situations you are confronted with will become increasing ambiguous and difficult to navigate.

It is for this reason that nursing schools and preceptor programs start with the basics and work up to more complex situations. As a new nurse it is nearly impossible to NOT focus simply on the tasks. That is fine as you are learning the basics but as you grow and progress you will find that your thinking will evolve and you will see things that you would have never noticed just months earlier.

Lastly, I want to make sure you fully understand that this is not a complete guide to every decision you will make in your career.

There are many things you can do to improve the efficiency and speed at which you are able to complete tasks. This is simply a base framework to help you make the base decisions required.

It has been observed that individuals make as many as 35,000 decisions a day. As a nurse that number is no doubt much higher. With so many decisions to make we run the risk of encountering a phenomena called "decision fatigue"

Decision Fatigue

In a <u>New York Times article decision fatigue</u>[2] is explained as such:

"No matter how rational and high-minded you try to be, you can't make decision after decision without paying a biological price. It's different from ordinary physical fatigue — you're not consciously aware of being tired — but you're low on mental energy. The more choices you make throughout the day, the harder each one becomes for your brain, and eventually it looks for shortcuts, usually in either of two very different ways."

We cannot make unlimited decisions without suffering the consequences of eventually making poor choices.

This priority framework is intended to take the decision out of the situation in essence, allowing you to focus on the patient and the immediate need.

On our podcast "NRSNG" and "Med of the Day" we often discuss priority issues and I share some of my experiences with tough choices.

You can do this. Do not be too hard on yourself as you work through figuring out how to make appropriate decisions in nursing. Prioritization can be learned as you begin to grasp the bigger picture.

1. GILLESPIE, M., & PATERSON, B. (2009). Helping Novice Nurses Make Effective Clinical Decisions: The Situated Clinical Decision-Making Framework. *Nursing Education Perspectives, 30*(3), 164-170. Retrieved February 23, 2015, from https://www.sjcme.edu/files/sjcme_files/docs/nursing/help-nurses-clinical-decisions.pdf

2. Tierney, J. (2011, August 20). Do You Suffer From Decision Fatigue? Retrieved February 23, 2015, from http://www.nytimes.com/2011/08/21/magazine/do-you-suffer-from-decision-fatigue.html?pagewanted=all&_r=0

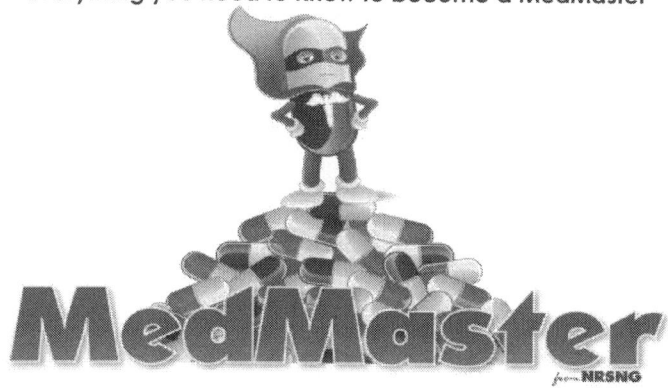

NCLEX® Essentials - Med Surg
Everything You Need to Know for the NCLEX®

NRSNG.com | NursingStudentBooks.com

Jon Haws RN CCRN
Tarang Patel RN CCRN SRNA
Sandra Haws RD CNSC MS

©**TazKai LLC** NRSNG.com First Edition July 2015

NCLEX® Essentials
MED SURG

The NCLEX® Doesn't
Have to be so
DAMN Hard!

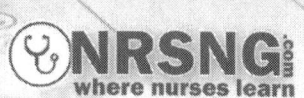

Introduction

While every NCLEX® exam is different by nature of computer adaptive testing, this book contains the most important information that will not only aid you in taking the exam, but also in your work as a nurse.

The purpose of this book is to condense the information you need to know into an easy to study and digest format. This is not a complete guide to Med-Surg (that is what text books are for) but rather an attempt to extract only the most vital information.

You should consult this book to review and highlight information as you work your way through nursing school and as you prepare for the NCLEX®.

Many students state that nursing school is "like drinking from a fire hose" . . . I would have to agree with that sentiment. I remember my time in nursing school, not only are you learning how to care for patients but you are learning new skills, a tremendous amount of new information, and essentially a new language . . . it's tough to say the least.

Our goal at NRSNG.com is to simplify your journey. You will still need to put in a huge amount of work, but we think that nursing school can be easier as you learn what exactly you should focus on and forget the fluff.

Enjoy the book. . .

Happy Nursing!

-Jon Haws RN BSN CCRN
CEO NRSNG.com

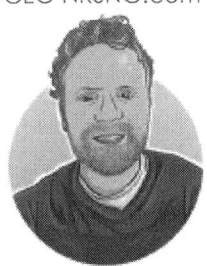

Cardiovascular Disorders

Cardiac Dysrhythmias

	Route			Rate	Rhythm	
Rhythm	P Wave	PR Interval	QRS	Rate	Regularity	Causes
Normal Sinus	Normal	0.12-0.20	<0.12	60-100	Regular	Normal Finding
Sinus Bradycardia	Normal	0.12-0.20	<0.12	<60	Regular	Sleep, inactivity, athletic, vagal tone, drugs, MI, K+, respiratory arrest
Sinus Tachycardia	Normal	0.12-0.20	<0.12	>100, usually 100-150	Regular	Caffeine, exercise, fever, anxiety, heart failure, drugs, pain, hypoxia, hypotension, volume depletion
Atrial Pause	Looks like SR but drops a complex			Normal or	Irregular	Elderly, digoxin toxicity

				slow		, MI, rheumatic fever
Atrial Flutter	Saw tooth	None	<0.12	Atrial rate 250-400	Regular or Irregular	Valvular heart disease, MI, CHF, pericarditis
Atrial Fibrillation	Wavy unidentifiable	None	<0.12	Atrial rate >400	Irregular	Heart disease, pulmonary disease, emotional stress, excessive alcohol or caffeine
Junctional Rhythm	INVERTED before or after QRS or absent	<0.12	<0.12	40-60	Regular	Electrical impulse not arriving from SA node, AV node fires at inherent rate
Accelerate	INVE	<0.12	<0.12	60-	Regula	Digoxin

Rhythm	P wave	PR	QRS	Rate	Regularity	Causes
d Junctional Rhythm	RTED before or after QRS or absent			100	r	toxicity, damage to AV node
Junctional Tachycardia	INVERTED before or after QRS or absent	<0.12	<0.12	>100	Regular	Same as SVT
Supraventricular Tachycardia	Pointed or hidden in T	Immeasurable	<0.12	150-250	Regular	Caffeine, CHF, fatigue, hypoxia, mitral valve disease, altered pacemaker in heart
Idioventricular Rhythm	None	None	>0.11 wide and bizarre	20-40	Regular	Digoxin toxicity, acute MI
Ventricular Tachycardia	None	None	>0.11 wide and	150-250	Regular	MI, ischemia,

				bizarre		digoxin toxicity, hypoxia, acidosis, ↓K+, ↓BP
Ventricular Fibrillation	None	None	None	None	Irregular, vary in size, shape and height	Follow PVC, VT, most common cause of sudden death
Asystole	Possible	None	None	None	No QRS	Follows VT/VFib, acidosis, hypoxia, ↓K+, hypothermia, drug overdose
1° AV Block	Normal	>0.20	<0.12	Varies	Regular or irregular	First sign of increasing AV block
2° AV Block Type I	Normal	Varies: progressively prolonged	<0.12	Varies	Regularly irregular: QRS dropp	Acute inferior MI, digoxin toxicity, vagal

					ed after progressively prolonged PRI	stimulation, conduction system disease
2° AV Block Type II	Normal	Consistent normal or prolonged	Normal or wide	Usually slow	Regular or irregular; occasionally dropped QRS	BBB, anterior MI, lesions of conduction system
3° AV Block	Normal	No relationship between PR & QRS	Wide	Slow	Regular	Atria and ventricles beat independently, digoxin or K+ toxicity, acute MI, ischemic heart disease
Premature Atrial Contractions	Yes, PAC P wave shaped different	May differ from underlying rhythm	<0.12	Rate of underlying rhythm	PAC complexes come early	Coffee, tea, alcohol, CHF, emotions, fatigue, fever,

						hypoxia, mitral valve disease
Premature Junctional Contractions	Inverted before or after QRS or absent	<0.12	<0.12	Rate of underlying rhythm	PJC make it irregular	Vagal tone, stress, caffeine, alcohol, heart failure, digoxin toxicity, ↓K+
Premature Ventricular Contractions	None	N/A	>0.11 wide and bizarre	Dependant on underlying rhythm	Irregular due to premature beat	Ventricular irritability, hypoxia, ↓K+, Ca, MI, digoxin toxicity, anxiety

Sinus Bradycardia

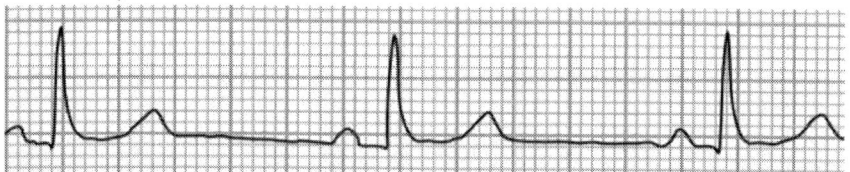

Sinus bradycardia is essentially the result of the SA node initiating impulses at a slower rate than normal. Conduction follows the correct path but at a slower rate.

1. Overview
   a. Rhythm is regular

b. Rate <60
2. NCLEX® Points
    a. Therapeutic Management
        i. Determine cause
        ii. Atropine may be administered to keep the rate >60
        iii. Monitor hemodynamics, insure proper CO
        iv. permanent pacemaker may be required

Premature Ventricular Contractions (PVC's)

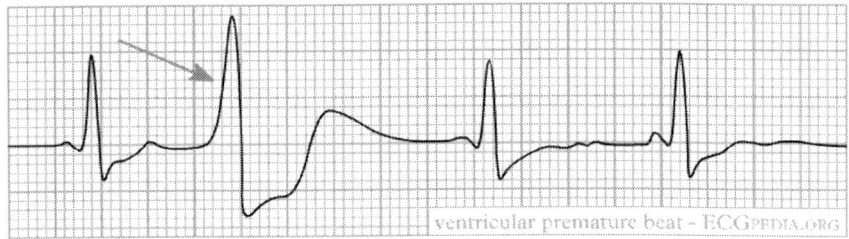

ventricular premature beat - ECGPEDIA.ORG

1. Overview
    a. early ventricular beats due to irritable ventricles
    b. may occur in repetitive pattern (bigeminy, trigemeny, quadrigeminy)
2. NCLEX® Points
    a. Therapeutic Management
        i. determine cause
        ii. assess for hypoxia
        iii. assess potassium level
        iv. notify physician if client complains of pain, increased frequency, R on T, multifocal

Ventricular Tachycardia

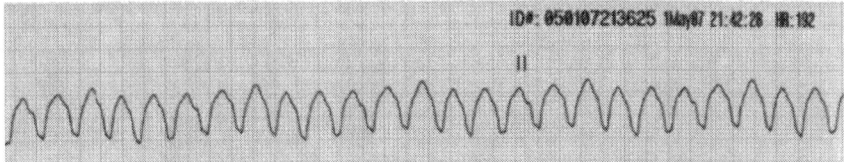

1. Overview

          a. irritable ventricles leas to repetitive firing of the
             ventricles
          b. may lead to cardiac arrest
    2. NCLEX® Points
          a. ASSESS for pulse first
              i. Pulse
                   1. Administer O2
                   2. Administer antidysrhythimcs
                   3. notify physician
                   4. cardioversion may be required
             ii. No Pulse
                   1. Begin ACLS protocol

Ventricular Fibrillation

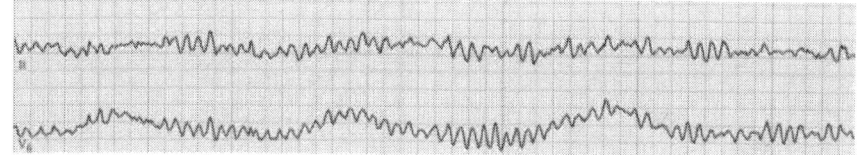

1. Overview
    a. ventricles quiver due to multiple irritable foci
    b. no cardiac output
    c. lethal rhythm
2. NCLEX® Points
    a. Therapeutic Interventions
        i. Begin ACLS protocol immediately
       ii. assess pulse and rhythm after 2 minutes of
           compressions

Myocardial Infarction

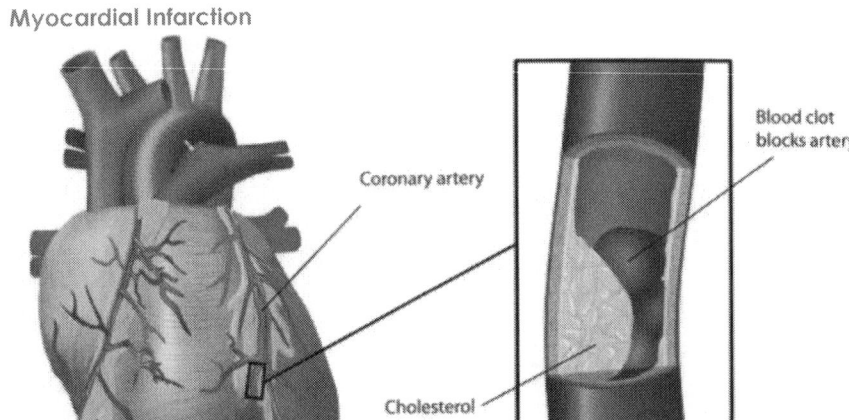

Coronary artery

Blood clot blocks artery

Cholesterol plaque buildup

Healthy heart muscle   Dead heart muscle

1. Overview
    a. Sudden restriction of blood supply to a portion of the heart.
2. NCLEX® Points
    a. Modifiable risk factors
        i. smoking
        ii. obesity
        iii. stress
        iv. ↑Chol
        v. Diabetes
        vi. HTN
    b. Angina Pectoris: chest pain due to restricted blood flow
        i. Stable angina: predictable with increased activity
        ii. Unstable angina: at rest and with activity
        iii. Prinzmetal angina: caused by vasospasm
    c. Nursing Assessment
        i. Chest pain unrelieved by rest
        ii. Crushing chest pain, diaphoresis, mottled skin, nausea, anxiety, SOB, palpitations

        iii. ST elevation on 12-lead

        iv. Elevated Troponins (most sensitive), elevated CK-MB

   d. Treatment

       i. MONA

          1. morphine, oxygen, nitroglycerin, aspirin

               a. Morphine - relieve chest pain

               b. Oxygen - increase oxygenation

               c. Nitrates - dilate coronary vessels - increase blood supply

               d. Aspirin - antiplatelet

       ii. Monitor EKG

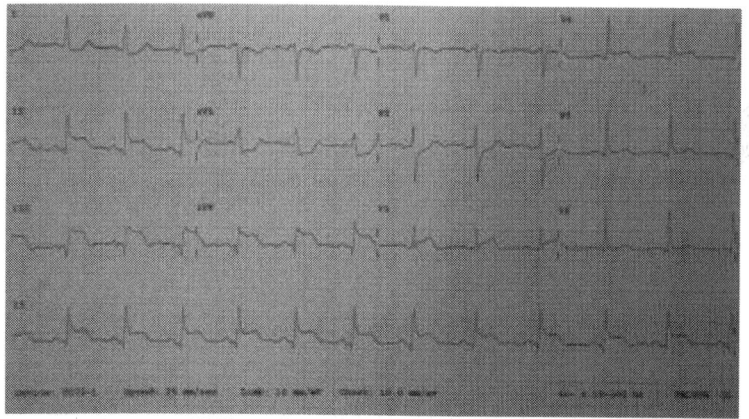

ST Elevation MI
By James Heilman, MD (Own work) [CC BY-SA 4.0 (http://creativecommons.org/licenses/by-sa/4.0)], via Wikimedia Commons

       iii. Rest - decrease O2 demands of heart

Heart Failure

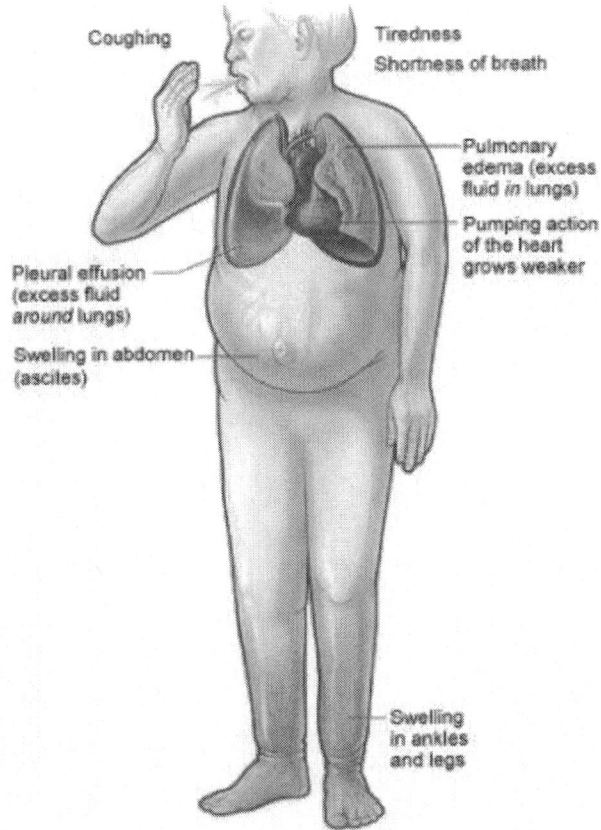

Coughing

Tiredness
Shortness of breath

Pulmonary
edema (excess
fluid *in* lungs)

Pumping action
of the heart
grows weaker

Pleural effusion
(excess fluid
around lungs)

Swelling in abdomen
(ascites)

Swelling
in ankles
and legs

1. Overview
    a. Heart is unable to pump enough blood to the
       body. Any condition that affects the hearts
       ability to pump can lead to Heart Failure (MI,
       valve disorders, HTN, pulmonary HTN).
    b. Initially presents as Right or Left side as it
       progresses both sides are affected.
    c. **Left Side**
        i. Left ventricle is unable to pump blood
           into the systemic circulation causing a
           "back-up" into the pulmonary circulation.
    d. **Right Side**

               i. Right ventricle is unable to pump blood into the pulmonary circulation causing a "back-up" in venous circulation.

2. NCLEX® Points
   a. Nursing Care
      i. raise head of bed
      ii. administer O2
      iii. Assess lung sounds
      iv. Encourage rest
      v. Monitor daily weights
      vi. Instruct on low sodium diet
   b. Medical Management
      i. Diuretics
      ii. Digoxin - improve contractility (CO) (assess apical pulse for 1 full minute)
      iii. ACE Inhibitors - decrease afterload (increase CO)

Right-Sided Failure	Left-Sided Failure
Systemic circulation	Pulmonary circulation
Dependent edema	Dyspnea
JVD	Crackles in lungs
Abdominal distention	Tachypnea

Valve Disorders
1. Overview
   a. Valves do not open (stenosis) or close (regurgitation) completely
   b. blood flow is jeopardized
2. NCELX® Points
   a. Types
      i. Mitral Stenosis
         1. mitral valve does not open completely during diastole
      ii. Mitral regurgitation
         1. Mitral valve does not close completely before systole

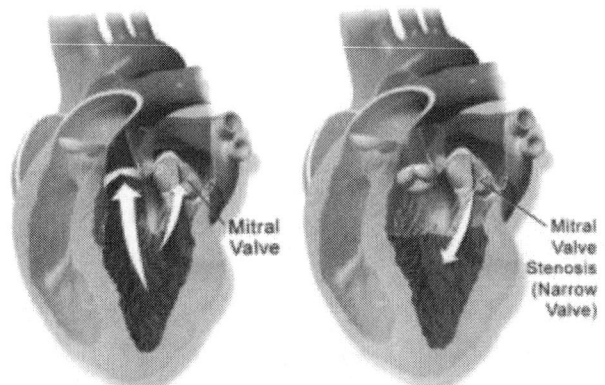

Mitral Valve Regurgitation   **Mitral Valve Stenosis**

    iii. Aortic Stenosis
       1. aortic valve does not open completely during systole
    iv. Aortic Regurgitation
       1. aortic valve does not close completely prior to diastole

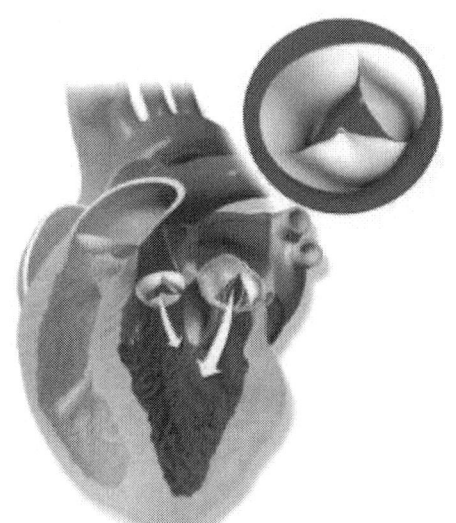

Aortic Regurgitation

Blausen.com staff. "Blausen gallery 2014". Wikiversity Journal of Medicine. DOI:10.15347/wjm/2014.010. ISSN 20018762. (Own work) [CC BY 3.0 (http://creativecommons.org/licenses/by/3.0)], via Wikimedia Commons

    b. Therapeutic Management

        i. Balloon valvuloplasty

        ii. Valve replacement

            1. Mechanical: lifetime anticoagulant therapy indicated

            2. Biological: valve from other species

            3. post op

                a. monitor hemodynamics

                b. monitor for signs of bleeding

                c. maintain good oral hygiene with soft bristle tooth brush

                d. prophylactic antibiotics required prior to invasive procedures

                e. instruct client on anticoagulant therapy

> f. avoid dental
>   procedures for 6 months

Endocarditis

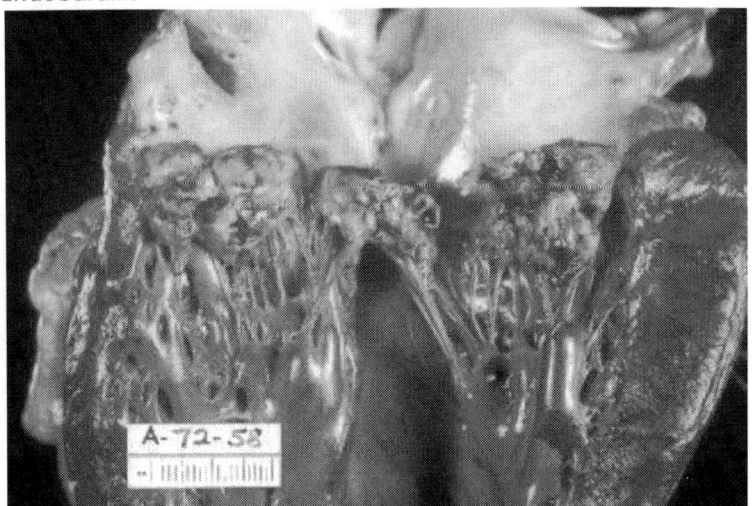

Mitral valve vegetation caused by bacterial endocarditis

1. Overview
    a. inflammation of the inner lining of the heart and valves
    b. common causes include IV drug use and valve replacement
    c. **Vegetations** form which are masses of platelets, fibrin, microorganisms, and inflammatory cells
        i. vegetations can become embolic
    d. infecting organism enters via:
        i. oral cavity (higher risk with recent dental procedure)
        ii. invasive procedures
        iii. infections
2. NCLEX® Points
    a. Assessment
        i. spiking fever
        ii. signs of heart failure
        iii. elevated WBC
        iv. heart murmurs
        v. Embolic complications from vegetations

1. Splinter hemorrhages in nail beds
2. Janeway lesions on fingers, toes, nose
3. Clubbing of fingers
b. Therapeutic Management
    i. Antiembolic stockings
    ii. IV antibiotic therapy
    iii. Oral hygiene with soft bristled tooth brush twice a day and rinse
    iv. Teach client to monitor for signs of infection
    v. Monitor for signs of emboli
    vi. Instruct dental provider of condition (prophylactic antibiotics needed)

Pericarditis

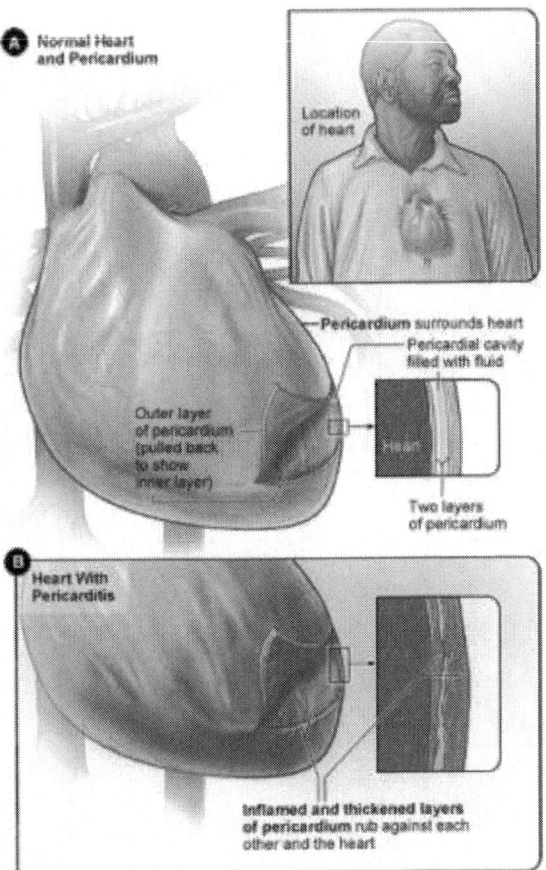

1. Overview
   a. inflammation of the pericardium
   b. compression of the heart occurs as the pericardial sac inflames
   c. heart failure or cardiac tamponade can occur
2. NCLEX® Points
   a. Assessment
      i. Pain
         1. chest radiating to left side of neck, shoulder, or back
         2. aggravated by inspiration, coughing, and swallowing

                3. worse in supine position, relieved by leaning forward
        ii. ST elevation
        iii. Signs of heart failure
    b. Therapeutic Management
        i. assess and treat pain
        ii. administer O2 and place client in high Fowler's
        iii. Assess for cardiac tamponade
                1. pulsus paradoxus (abnormally large decrease in systolic blood pressure and pulse wave amplitude during inspiration)
                2. JVD with clear lungs
                3. narrow pulse pressure (difference between SBP and DBP)
                4. Decreased CO
                5. Muffled heart sounds
                6. For more information on Cardiac Tamponade visit: http://goo.gl/umTsKA

Hypertension
    1. Overview
        a. SBP >140 or >90 DBP based on average of three separate readings
        b. Classified in stages
            i. Visit Mayo Clinic for more information on stages: http://goo.gl/icZSxe
    2. NCLEX Points
        a. Assessment
            i. past cardiovascular, cerebrovascular, renal, or thyroid disease, diabetes, smoking, alcohol use.
            ii. family history
            iii. referred to as silent killer as asymptomatic until end organ damage occurs
        b. Therapeutic Management

i. record I&O
ii. assess for cardiovascular changes
iii. weight reduction and lifestyle changes
iv. assess renal and neuro status
v. Medication therapy
    1. ACE Inhibitors
    2. Beta Blockers
    3. Calcium Channel Blockers
    4. Diuretics
vi. Lifestyle modifications
    1. Sodium restriction
    2. DASH diet
    3. smoking cessation
vii. Orthostatic hypotension: rapid drop in SBP of 10-20mmHg in upright position
    1. raise slowly
    2. avoid bathes and strenuous activity after taking medications
viii. Instruct pt to take medications even if asymptomatic

Cardiomyopathy

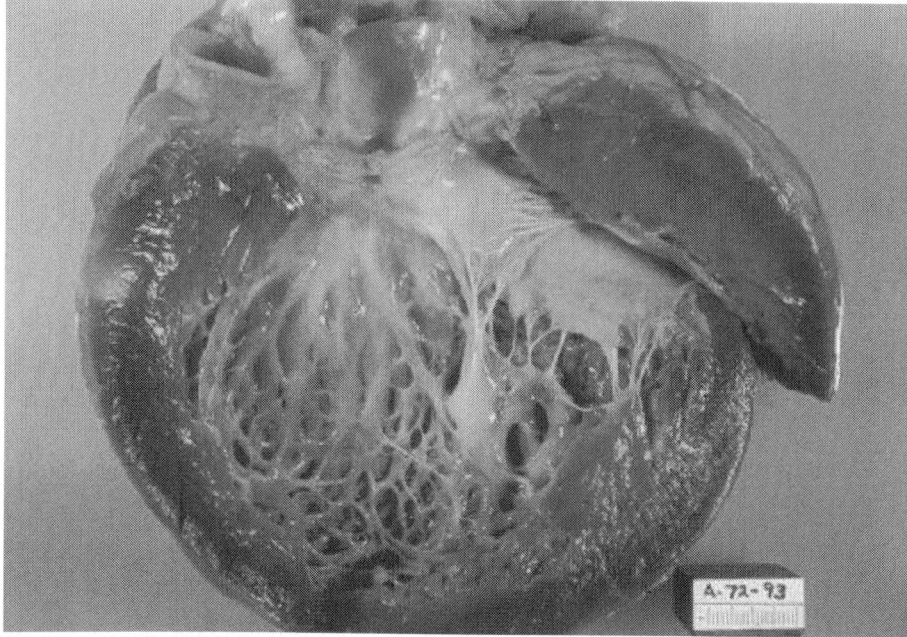

Thickened, dilated left ventricle

1. Overview
   a. Abnormality of heart muscle leading to functional changes
   b. Three types
      i. Dilated: all 4 chambers enlarged, ↓ contractility, ↓CO
      ii. Hypertrophic: progressive thickening of ventricular muscle, ↓CO
      iii. Restrictive: rigid ventricular walls do not stretch during filling, leads to right HF, ↓SV, ↓CO
2. NCLEX® Points
   a. Assessment
      i. fatigue (dyspnea)
      ii. dysrhythmias
      iii. extra heart sounds (s3 and s4)
   b. Therapeutic Management
      i. monitor for signs of HF
      ii. Encourage rest and minimize stress

Peripheral Arterial Disease

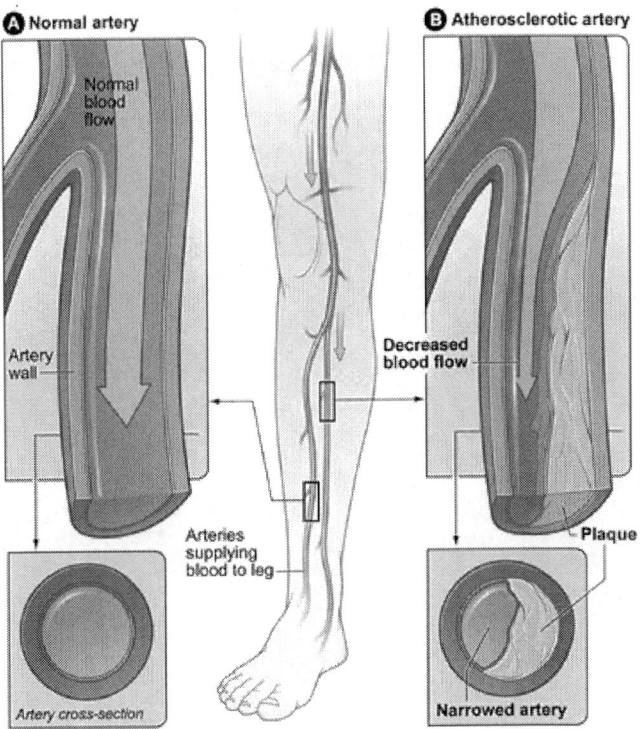

A Normal artery
B Atherosclerotic artery
Normal blood flow
Artery wall
Arteries supplying blood to leg
Artery cross-section
Decreased blood flow
Plaque
Narrowed artery

1. Overview
   a. Chronic arterial occlusion leads to decreased oxygen supply to lower extremities
   b. Atherosclerosis most common cause
2. NCLEX® Points
   a. Assessment
      i. Intermittent claudication (muscle pain following predictable amount of activity relieved by rest)
      ii. Rest pain which awakens the client from sleep
      iii. loss of hair on lower extremities
      iv. Cool, pale, numb extremities

b. Therapeutic Management
   i. assess pulses
   ii. smoking cessation
   iii. encourage exercise to the point of claudication then rest
   iv. Angioplasty
   v. Endarterectomy
   vi. Bypass grafting

Raynaud's Disease

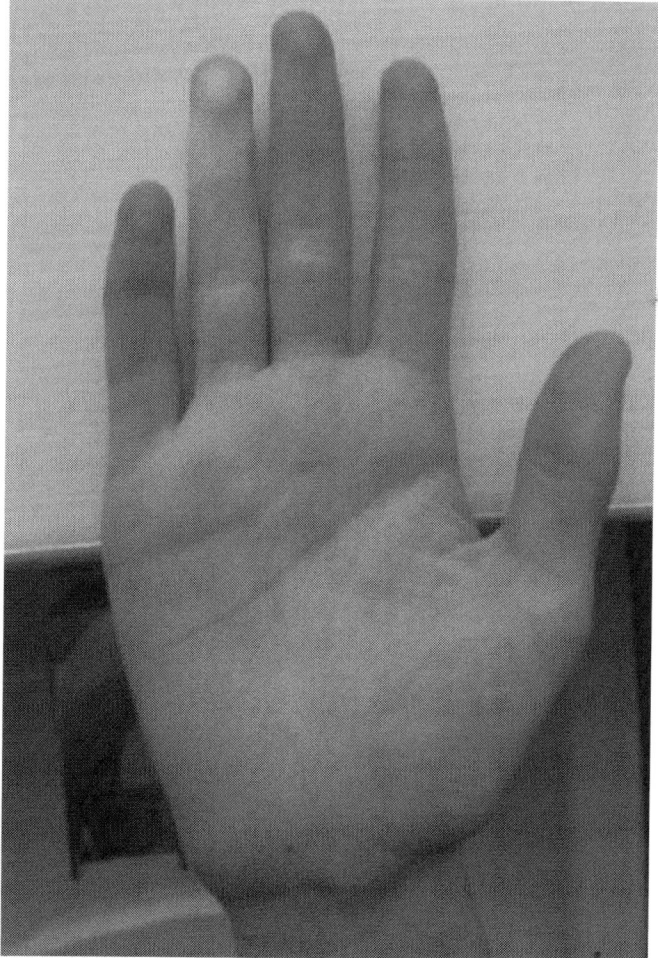

1. Overview
    a. Vasospasm of small arteries and arterioles of hands (less commonly feet, cheeks, ears)
    b. Occur when exposed to cold or stress
2. NCLEX® Points
    a. Assessment
        i. Triphasic color changes (pallor, cyanosis, rubor)
        ii. numbness, tingling, swelling
    b. Therapeutic Management
        i. identify and avoid precipitating factors
        ii. smoking cessation
        iii. wear warm clothing
        iv. medications
            1. analgesics
            2. vasodilators
            3. calcium channel blockers (vasospasm prevention)

Buerger's Disease (thromboangiitis obliterans)

1. Overview
    a. Inflammatory disease of the medium to small arteries and veins of the arms and legs
    b. microthrombi form and lead to vasospasm
2. NCLEX® Points
    a. Assessment
        i. Rest pain
        ii. Intermittent claudication
        iii. pain is most severe at night
        iv. diminished pulses
        v. ulceration in extremities
    b. Therapeutic Management
        i. smoking cessation
        ii. Medication
            1. Calcium channel blockers (prevent vasospasm)
            2. analgesics

        iii. Surgical treatment
              1. bypass grafting
              2. sympathectomy - surgical
                  dissection of nerve fibers

Aortic Aneurysm

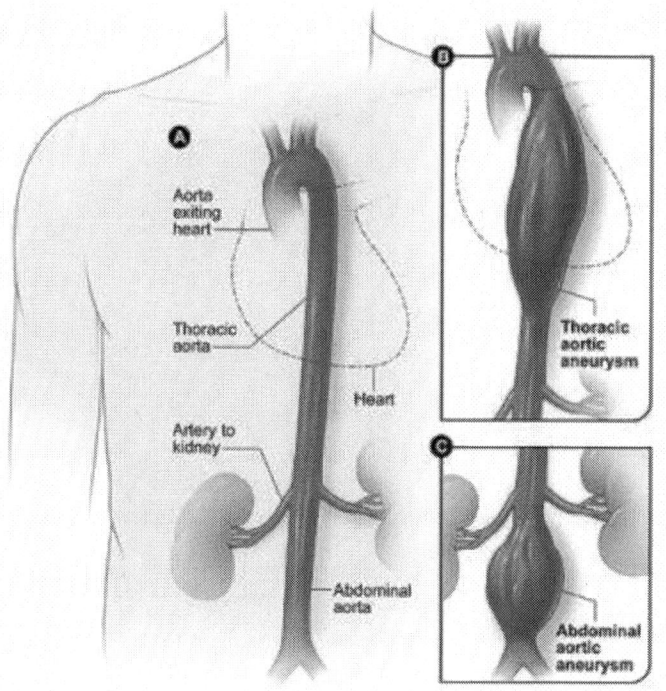

1. Overview
    a. dilation/out pouching of the aorta due to
        weakened medial layer
    b. classified by location
            i. thoracic
            ii. abdominal
    c. types
            i. dissecting: blood vessels separated by
                layer of blood
            ii. fusiform: dilation that involves the entire
                 circumference
            iii. saccular: localized out pouching

                    iv. false: clot forms outside the vessel wall
    2. NCLEX® Points
        a. Assessment
            i. thoracic
                1. pain in back, shoulders, abdomen
                2. dyspnea
            ii. abdominal
                1. pulsating mass in the abdomen
                2. systolic bruit
                3. tenderness on abdominal palpation
                4. hematoma on flank
            iii. Rupture assessment
                1. severe sudden onset of pain
                2. pain radiating to flank and groin
                3. signs of shock
        b. Therapeutic Management
            i. Reduce blood pressure
            ii. diagnose via CT or abdominal ultrasound
            iii. Abdominal aortic aneurysm resection/EVAR (endovascular aneurysm repair)
                1. assess peripheral pulses
                2. monitor renal function (due to blood loss and decreased perfusion)
                    a. urine output, renal labs
                3. assess vital signs
                4. assess incision site

Thrombophlebitis
    1. Overview
        a. thromubs (clot) formation with associated inflammation
        b. Virchow's Triad
            i. Venous stasis
            ii. Damage to inner lining of vein
            iii. Hypercoagulability of blood

        c. Risk for pulmonary embolism if detachment occurs

2. NCLEX® Points
    a. Assessment
        i. Risk factors
            1. history of thrombophlebitis, pelvic surgery, obesity, HF, a-fib, immobility, MI, pregnancy, IV therapy, hypercoagulabiity
        ii. Assessment findings
            1. unilateral edema
            2. pain
            3. warm skin
            4. febrile state
            5. Homan's sign - pain on dorsiflexion of foot
        iii. Therapeutic management
            1. analgesia
            2. ultrasound to confirm finding
            3. monitor respiratory status
                a. report pink sputum, tachypnea, tachycardia, chest pain (signs of pulmonary embolism)
            4. monitor circumference of affected limb
            5. monitor distal pulses
            6. smoking cessation
            7. avoid long periods of sitting
            8. elevate legs 10-20 min every few hours
            9. monitor PT and INR for patients on Coumadin (warfarin)
            10. monitor PTT for patients on Heparin therapy

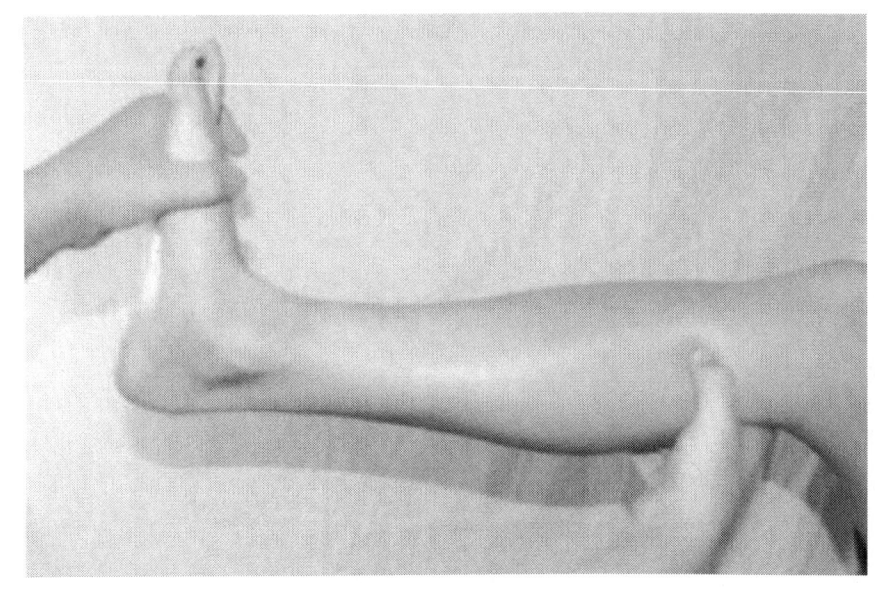

1. Heart Rate
    a. normal sinus 60-100bpm
    b. sinus tachycardia >100bpm
    c. sinus bradycardia <60bpm
2. Vascular System
    a. arteries
        i. carry oxygenated blood to tissues
    b. veins
        i. carry deoxygenated blood back to heart
3. Cardiac Markers
    a. Indication of cardiac damage

Troponin	Most sensitive to cardiac damage	12 hours
CK-MB	Sensitive when skeletal damage isn't present	10-24 hours
Myoglobin (Mb)	Low specificity to infarction	2 hours

4. Labs
    a. Potassium
        i. Hypokalemia
            1. ventricular dysrhythmias
            2. ↑ digoxin toxicity
            3. U wave
            4. ST depression
        ii. Hyperkalemia
            1. Peaked T waves
            2. Wide QRS
            3. Ventricular dysrhythmias
    b. ↑ Hematocrit indicates volume depletion
    c. ↓Hematocrit and hemoglobin indicate anemia
    d. Lipids
        i. Total cholesterol ↓200 mg/dL
        ii. LDL ↓130 mg/dL
        iii. HDL 30-70 mg/dL
5. Holter monitoring provides 24 hour EKG monitoring

     a. client should record any moment that they have chest pain
6. Assess for iodine, seafood allergies prior to any dye tests
7. Cardiac Catheterization
     a. used to assess cardiac function (valve and chamber function)
     b. monitor distal pulses
     c. monitor pressure dressing and insertion site for bleeding or hematoma
8. Angioplasty
     a. used to dilate occluded cardiac vessels
     b. encourage fluid intake to flush dye from system
     c. assess distal pulses
9. Cardioversion
     a. synchronized to R wave
        i. if not synchronized shock could cause VF
10. Coronary artery disease
     a. narrowing of coronary arteries due to plaque build up
        i. may lead to MI, HF, HTN, angina
        ii. ST depression occurs with ischemia
     b. client should follow low fat, low cholesterol, high fiber diet
11. Vena Cava Filter
     a. assess cardiac, neuro, and respiratory status post op
     b. avoid hip flexion
     c. assess for bleeding and hematoma at insertion site
     d. assess peripheral pulses
     e. anti embolic stockings
     f. anti coagulant therapy
12. Cardiogenic Shock
     a. heart is unable maintain effective cardiac output
     b. Assessment
        i. low urine output
        ii. ↓BP
        iii. Assess CVP (pressure in superior vena cava representing right atrial pressure preload)
           1. CVP: 2-8 mmHg

2. reading should be taken at end expiration if ventilated
3. Zero transducer at the fourth intercostal space along the mid axillary line (location of the right atrium)

Respiratory Disorders

Asthma

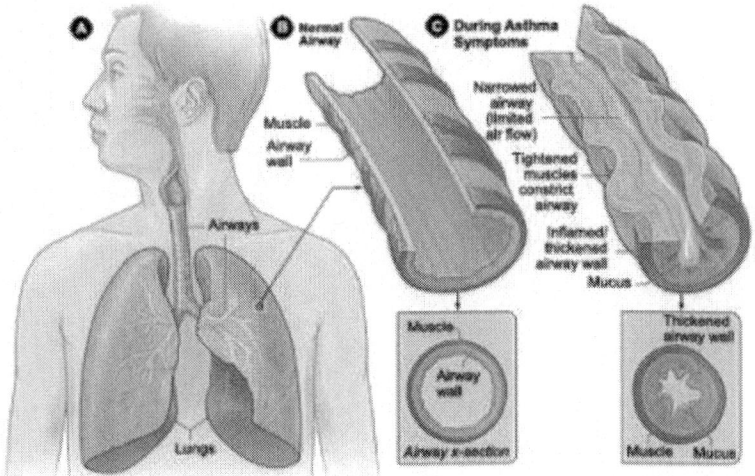

1. Overview
   a. Inflammatory disorder of the airways stimulated by triggers (infection, allergens, exercise, irritant)
   b. Status asthmaticus is a life-threatening condition unresponsive to treatment
2. NCLEX® Points
   a. Assessment
      i. wheezing/crackles
      ii. restlessness
      iii. diminished breath sounds
      iv. tachypnea
   b. Therapeutic Management
      i. High Fowler's position
      ii. Administer O2
      iii. Administer bronchodilators BEFORE corticosteroids

Chronic Obstructive Pulmonary Disease (COPD)

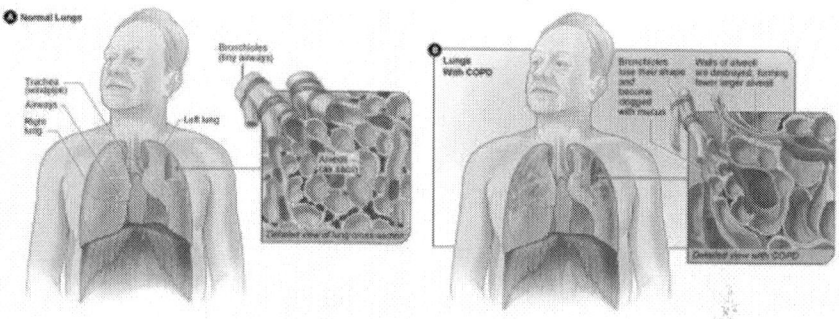

1. Overview
    a. Obstruction of airflow due to emphysema and chronic bronchitis
        i. emphysema
            1. destruction of alveoli due to chronic inflammation
            2. decreased surface area for gas exchange
        ii. chronic bronchitis
            1. chronic airway inflammation with productive cough
            2. excessive sputum production
2. NCLEX® Points
    a. Assessment
        i. Barrel chest
        ii. use of accessory muscles
        iii. congestion on chest Xray
        iv. ABG with ↑CO_2 and ↓pH (respiratory acidosis)
    b. Therapeutic Management
        i. Do not administer O2 at greater than 2 L/min
            1. stimulus to breath is low Po2 not elevated Pco2 (as in healthy individuals)
            2. assess SpO2
            3. provide chest physiotherapy (CPT)
            4. teach pursed lip breathing

5. avoid allergens and triggers (dust, infections, spicy foods, smoking)
6. Increase fluid intake to 3000 mL/day to keep secretions thin
7. small frequent meals to prevent hypoxia

Pneumothorax and Hemothorax

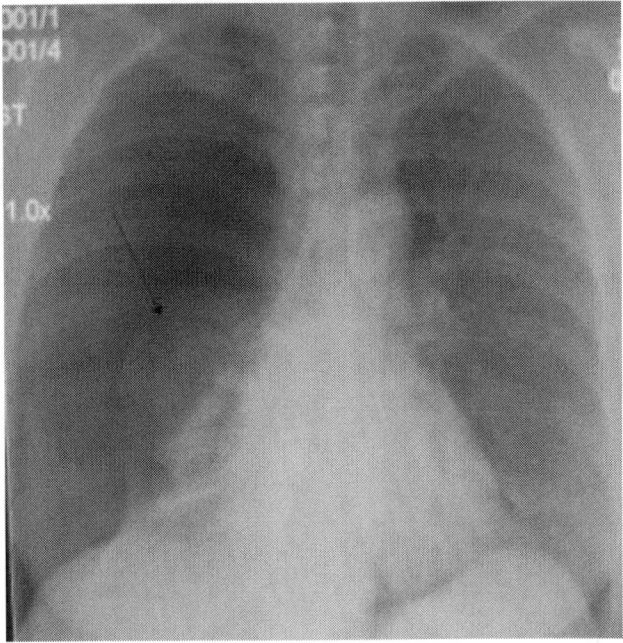

1. Overview
   a. Pneumothorax
      i. Spontaneous: ruptured bleb on lung surface fills pleural space compressing lung (collapsed lung)
         1. primary: rupture of bleb in otherwise healthy individual
         2. secondary: rupture of distended alveoli may occur with COPD
      ii. Tension: injury to chest wall leading to shift in mediastinum to unaffected side and disruption of venous return to the

heart. This is a medical emergency due to severely compromised cardiac output and building pressure in chest cavity.
   b. Hemothorax
       i. Blood accumulation in pleural space
2. NCLEX® Points
    a. Assessment
        i.   Decreased or absent breath sounds on affected side
        ii. decreased chest expansion on affected side
        iii. tracheal deviation to unaffected side (tension pneumothorax)
        iv. Dullness (hemothorax)
        v.   dyspnea
        vi. hyperresonance (pneumothorax)
    b. Therapeutic Management
        i.   chest tube insertion
        ii. thoracentesis
        iii. high Fowler's position
        iv. Open pneumothorax
             1. if the pneumothorax is due to an open (sucking) chest wound the hole should be covered immediately with a nonporous (occlusive) dressing sealed on three sides. This prevents air from entering during inhalation while allowing it to escape during expiration.

Main symptoms of infectious
Pneumonia

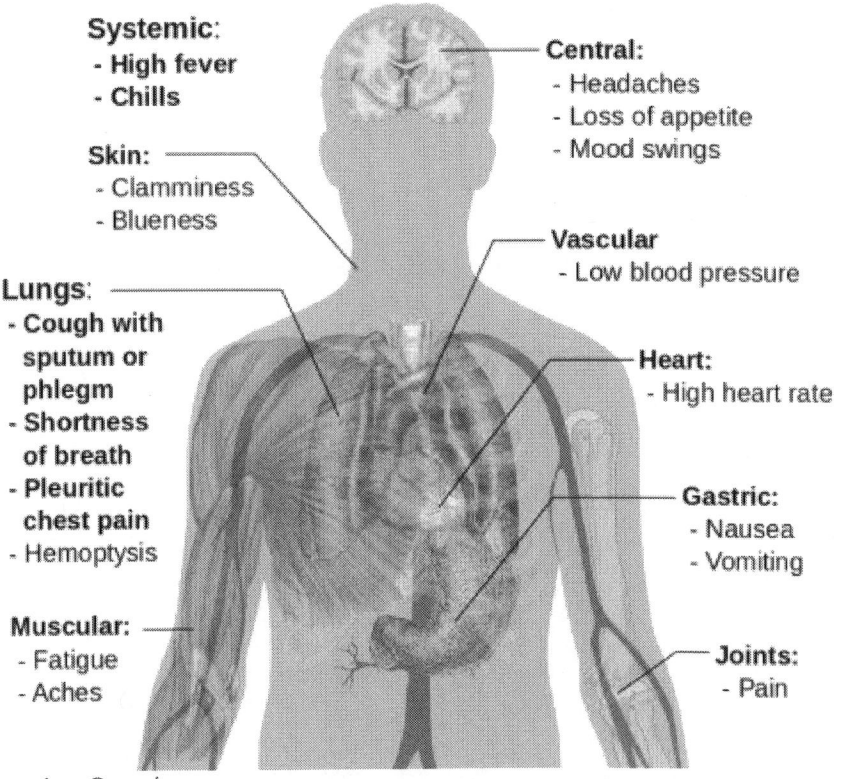

Systemic:
- **High fever**
- **Chills**

Skin:
- Clamminess
- Blueness

Lungs:
- **Cough with sputum or phlegm**
- **Shortness of breath**
- **Pleuritic chest pain**
- Hemoptysis

Muscular:
- Fatigue
- Aches

Central:
- Headaches
- Loss of appetite
- Mood swings

Vascular
- Low blood pressure

Heart:
- High heart rate

Gastric:
- Nausea
- Vomiting

Joints:
- Pain

1. Overview
    a. Inflammatory condition of the lungs primarily affecting the alveoli which may fill with fluid or pus.
    b. Infectious vs Noninfectious
        i.   infectious
            1. bacterial vs viral
        ii. non infectious
            1. aspiration
    c. Community acquired vs Hospital acquired vs Opportunistic
    d. Chest Xray and Sputum culture necessary
    e. sputum culture identifies organism

2. NCLEX® Points
    a. Assessment
        i. Viral
            1. low grade fever
            2. non productive cough
            3. WBCs normal to low elevation
            4. Chest X-ray shows minimal changes
            5. less severe than bacterial
        ii. Bacterial
            1. high fever
            2. productive cough
            3. WBCs elevated
            4. Chest X-ray shows infiltrates
            5. more severe
    b. NCLEX® Points
        i. Assessment
            1. As above
            2. chills
            3. rhonchi and wheezes
            4. sputum production
        ii. Therapeutic Management
            1. antibiotics, analgesics, antipyretics
            2. supplemental O2
            3. maintain airway and assess respiratory status
            4. encourage activity as soon as possible
            5. instruct on chest expansion exercises, coughing and deep breathing
            6. obtain vaccinations for influenza and pneumococcal pneumonia
            7. proper hand hygiene
            8. encourage 3 L/day of fluids unless contraindicated

Tuberculosis
    1. Overview

a. Lung infection causing pneumonitis and granulomas in the lungs
b. Noncompliance with treatment may lead to drug resistance (MDR-TB)
c. Transmission caused by airborn route via droplets

2. NCLEX® Points
   a. When contact with an infected individual occurs chest x-ray and skin test are completed
   b. Risk of transmission is reduced after 2-3 weeks of medication regimen
   c. Assessment
      i. Night sweats
      ii. Chills
      iii. Fatigue
      iv. Weight loss
      v. Persistent cough
   d. Client history
      i. Foreign travel
      ii. Living in tight quarters
      iii. Past exposure
      iv. Sputum cultures
   e. Therapeutic Management
      i. Place in a negative pressure room
      ii. Skin test should be measured in size
      iii. Particulate respirator must be worn
      iv. Isoniazide, pyrazinamide and rifampin
      v. Treatment should continue for 6-12 months

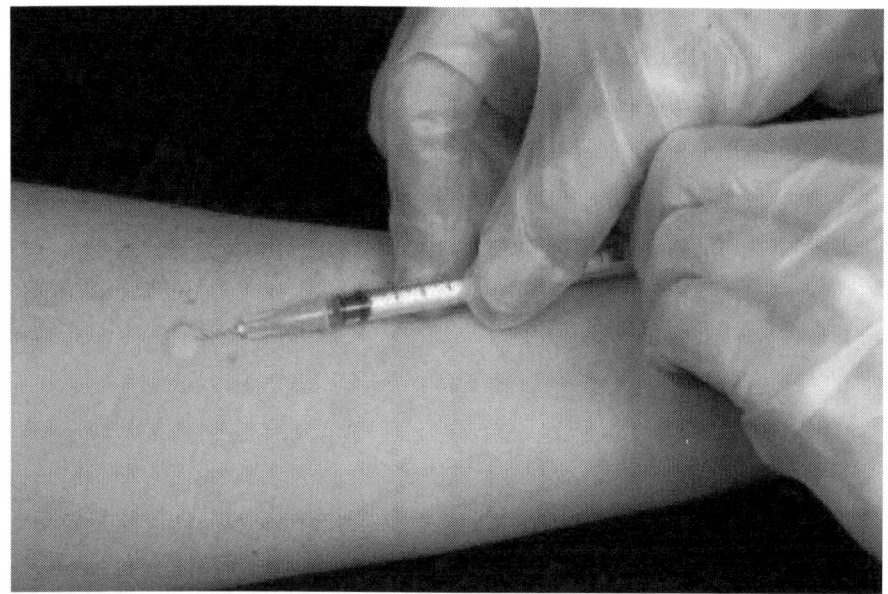

Pulmonary Embolism (PE)
1. Overview
   a. Emboli in pulmonary circulation block blood flow to pulmonary capillaries
   b. Common causes
      i. immobilization
      ii. long bone fractures
      iii. hypercoagulabiity
      iv. DVT in large veins
   c. Gas exchange is impaired leading to pulmonary infarction
2. NCLEX® Points
   a. Assessment
      i. VQ scan (ventilation perfusion scan) used to diagnose
      ii. Low PaO2
      iii. restlessness, anxiety
      iv. Tachycardia, tachypnea, hypotension, fever
      v. Altered LOC
      vi. diaphoresis and cyanosis
   b. Therapeutic Management
      i. O2 therapy
      ii. prepare for ventilation

        iii.   Anticoagulant

        iv.   Analgesics

        v.   Vena cava filter insertion

NCLEX® Cram - Respiratory

1. Sputum culture
    a. obtain sample prior to beginning antibiotic therapy
2. Keep client NPO post bronchoscopy until gag reflex returns
3. Thoracentesis

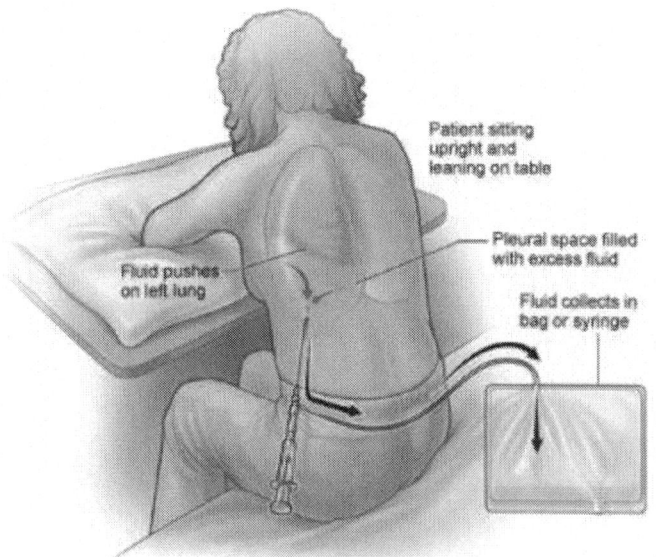

Patient sitting upright and leaning on table

Pleural space filled with excess fluid

Fluid collects in bag or syringe

Fluid pushes on left lung

    a. position the client sitting upright leaning forward onto a bedside table with arms supporting weight
    b. monitor for pneumothorax and PE

4. Lung Biopsy - Post Procedure
    a. monitor sight for drainage and bleeding
    b. monitor respiratory status and assess for signs of pneumothorax
5. Normal ABG Values
    a. pH: 7.35 - 7.45
    b. PCO2: 35-45 mmHg

     c. HCO3: 22-26 mEq/L
     d. PO2: 80-100 mmHg
     e. SpO2: 96%-100%
     f.   Acedemia = pH <7.35
     g. Alkalemia = pH>7.45

6. SpO2: % of O2 bound to hemoglobin compared to total HgB capable of binding)
     a. remove nail polish
     b. poor circulation will diminish accuracy

7. Hierarchy of O2 Delivery

Method

Nasal Cannula
1 lpm = 24%
2 lpm = 28%
3 lpm = 32%
4 lpm = 36%
5 lpm = 40%
6 lpm = 44%

Simple Face Mask
5 lpm = 40%
6 lpm = 45-50%
7 lpm = 50-55%
8 lpm = 55-60%

Non-rebreather Mask
6 lpm = 60%
7 lpm = 70%
8 lpm = 80%
9 lpm = 90%
10 lpm = close to 100%

Venturi Mask
4 lpm = 24-28%
8 lpm = 35-40%
12 lpm = 50%

Trach Collar
21-70% at 10L

T-Piece
21-100% with flow rate at 2.5 times minute ventilation

CPAP
Positive airway pressure during spontaneous breaths

Bi-PAP
Positive pressure during spontaneous breaths (IPAP) and preset pressure to be maintained during expiration (EPAP/PEEP)

SIMV

Preset Vt and f. Circuit remains open between mandatory breaths so pt can take additional breaths. Ventilator doesn't cycle during spontaneous breaths so Vt varies.
Mandatory breaths synchronized so they do not occur during spontaneous breaths.

Assist Control
Preset Vt and f and inspiratory effort required to assist spontaneous breaths.
Delivers control breaths. Cycles additionally if pt inspiratory effort is adequate.
Same Vt delivered for spontaneous breaths.

7. Ventilator Alarms
   a. High Pressure
      i. Kink in tubing
      ii. cough, gag, or biting tube
      iii. increased secretions
   b. Low Pressure
      i. ET tube disconnection
8. Rib fractures will cause pain during inspiration
9. Flail chest causes paradoxical respirations
10. Acute Respiratory Distress Syndrome (ARDS)
    a. ABG: respiratory acidosis (pH<7.35 CO_2>45 PaO_2 <80)
11. Tripod position and pursed lipped breathing helpful to COPD patients
12. Influenza
    a. vaccination recommended yearly for
       i. health care workers
       ii. elderly
       iii. children
       iv. immunocompromised
13. If a patient has an injured neck use chin thrust rather than head tilt to open airway
14. Limit airway suctioning to 10 seconds
15. Rotate catheter and use intermittent suction
16. Lung injury - Good Lung Down positioning
17. High fowlers (>45 degrees) positioning for respiratory failure patients
18. Mask should be worn at all times with droplet isolation
19. Pink Puffer vs Blue Bloater

a. Pink Puffer: emphysema
    i. barrel-shaped chest, hyperinflated chest, pursed lipped breathing
b. Blue Bloater: bronchitis
    i. hypoxia, obese, water retention, dependent on hypoxia for respiratory drive
20. Atelectisis: incomplete expansion or collapse of lung

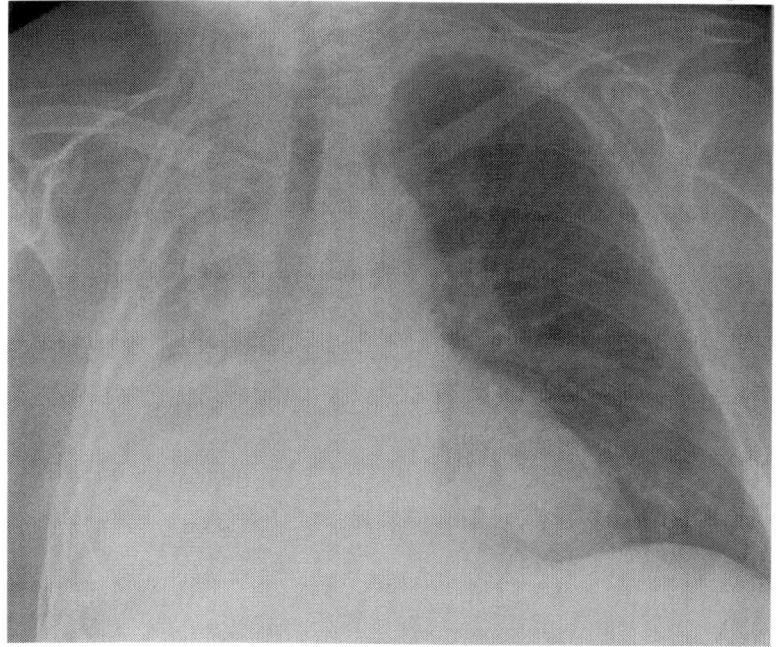

Increased Intracranial Pressure (ICP)

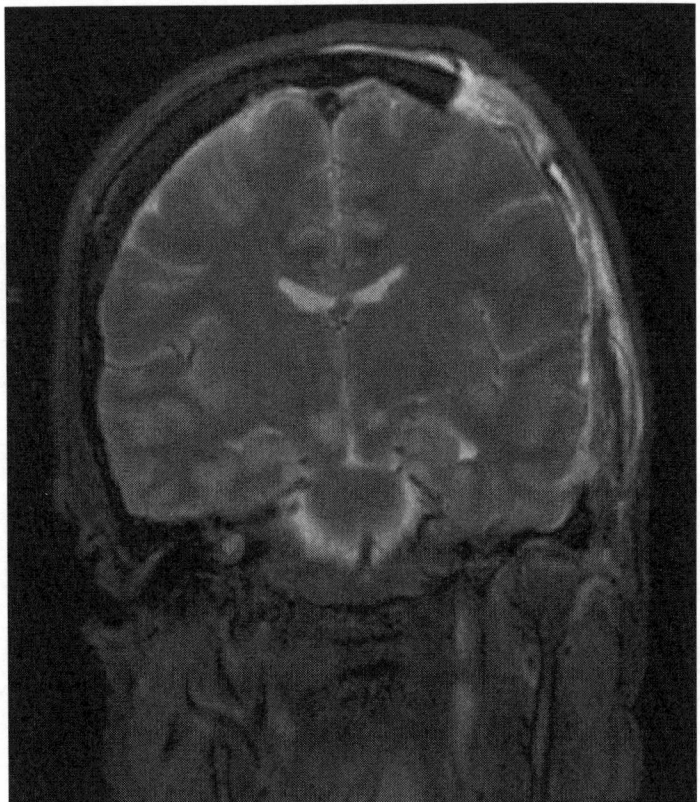

Increasing ICP can lead to brain herniation

1. Overview
   a. Normal ICP: 5-15mmHg
   b. ICP can elevate due to trauma, hemorrhage, tumor, hydrocephlaus, inflammation
   c. The cranial vault is rigid, increased ICP can limit cerebral perfusion, impeded CSF absorption and lead to herniation of brain tissue causing death
2. NCLEX® Points

a. Assessment

    i. Levels of Consciousness

Conscious	Normal	Assessment of LOC involves checking orientation: people who are able promptly and spontaneously to state their name, location, and the date or time are said to be oriented to self, place, and time, or "oriented X3". A normal sleep stage from which a person is easily awakened is also considered a normal level of consciousness. "Clouding of consciousness" is a term for a mild alteration of consciousness with alterations in attention and wakefulness.
Confused	Disoriented; impaired thinking and responses	People who do not respond quickly with information about their name, location, and the time are considered "obtuse" or "confused". A confused person may be bewildered, disoriented, and have difficulty following instructions. The person may have slow thinking and possible memory time loss. This could be caused by sleep deprivation, malnutrition, allergies, environmental pollution, drugs (prescription and nonprescription), and infection.
Delirious	Disoriented; restlessness, hallucinations, sometimes delusions	Some scales have "delirious" below this level, in which a person may be restless or agitated and exhibit a marked deficit in attention.
Somnolent	Sleepy	A *somnolent* person shows excessive drowsiness and responds to stimuli only with incoherent mumbles or disorganized movements.
Obtunded	Decreased alertness; slowed psychomotor responses	In *obtundation*, a person has a decreased interest in their surroundings, slowed responses, and sleepiness.

Stuporous	Sleep-like state (not unconscious); little/no spontaneous activity	People with an even lower level of consciousness, stupor, only respond by grimacing or drawing away from painful stimuli.
Comatose	Cannot be aroused; no response to stimuli	Cannot be aroused; no response to stimuli

       ii.   headache

      iii.   Cushing's Triad

           1.   abnormal respirations

           2.   widening pulse pressure

           3.   reflex bradycardia

      iv.   elevated temp

       v.   pupilary changes

      vi.   posturing

      vii.   seizures

     viii.   positive Babinski reflex

   b.   Therapeutic Management

       i.   monitory respiratory status

      ii.   monitor pupil changes

      iii.   avoid sedatives and CNS depressants

      iv.   Hypocapnia (PaCO2 30-35 mmHg) will lead to cerebral vasoconstriction leading to decreased ICP

       v.   monitor temperature

      vi.   prevent shivering

      vii.   decrease stimuli

     viii.   monitor electrolytes

      ix.   avoid Valsalva's maneuver

       x.   Ventricular drain and ICP monitoring

      xi.   Assess neuro status q 1-2 hours

      xii.   elevate HOB to at least 30 degrees

     xiii.   Osmotic diuretics and corticosteroids

Stroke

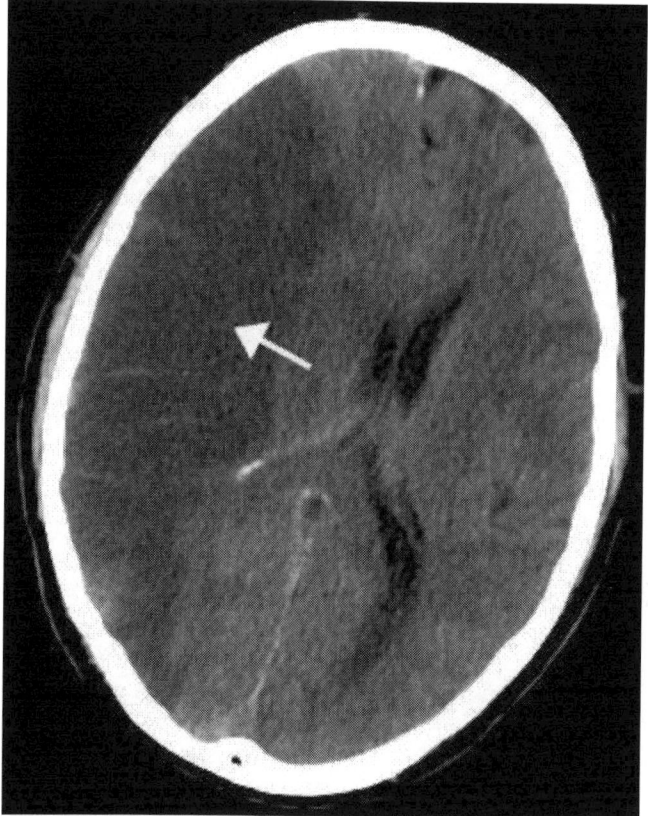

Right MCA Infarct

1. Overview
    a. Neurological deficit caused by decreased blood flow to a portion of the brain
    b. May be ischemic or hemorrhagic
    c. Lack of blood flow greater than 10 minutes can cause irreversible damage
    d. Risk factors:
        i.   HTN
        ii. Diabetes
        iii. atherosclerosis

            iv. cardiac dysrhythmias

            v. substance abuse

            vi. obesity

            vii. oral contraceptives

            viii. anticoagulant therapy

        e. Diagnosed via: CT, MRI, cerebral arteriogram (hemorrhagic and late ischemic)

2. NCLEX® Points

    a. Assessment

        i. contralateral manifestations (opposite side of stroke)

        ii. FAST

            1. facial droop

            2. arms - does one arm drift?

            3. speech problems

            4. time - call 9-1-1

        iii. dependent on location

            1. Aphasia - speech difficulty

                a. Expressive - understands but unable to communicate verbally

                b. Receptive - unable to comprehend spoke and written word

                c. Global - language dysfunction

                d. Interventions

                    i. provide adequate time for client to respond

                    ii. repeat names of individuals and objects frequently

                    iii. use a picture board

     iv. provide only
      one instruction
      at a time
   2. Apraxia - inability to perform
    tasks
   3. Hemianopsia - blindness in half
    the vision field
     a. instruct client to turn
      head to capture the
      entire vision field
     b. approach client from
      unaffected side
     c. provide food and
      objects to unaffected
      side
   4. Dysphagia - difficulty swallowing
 b. Therapeutic Management
   i. involve speech therapy
   ii. ischemic stroke
    1. permissive hypertension
    2. antithrombitic therapy
    3. carotid endartecomy
    4. thrombectomy
    5. monitor neurological status
   iii. hemorrhagic stroke
    1. coiling or clipping of aneurysm
    2. monitor neurological status
   iv. seizure precautions
   v. monitor level of consciousness
   vi. monitor neurological status
   vii. maintain quiet, calm environment
   viii. assess need for assistive devices
   ix. involve physical and occupational
    therapy

Seizure Disorder
View the NRSNG.com video on Seizures here:
https://youtu.be/lr2G34fl4Fg
1. Overview
   a. Abnormal excessive discharge of electrical activity in the brain
   b. Types
      i. Generalized - both hemispheres
         1. Tonic-clonic
         2. absence
         3. myoclonic
         4. atonic
      ii. Partial - one hemisphere
         1. simple partial
         2. complex partial
   c. Risk factors
      i. genetics
      ii. trauma
      iii. tumors
      iv. toxicity
      v. infection
      vi. cerebral bleeding or swelling
      vii. acute febrile state
   d. Status epilepticus - persistent seizure activity with little or no break
2. NCLEX® Points
   a. Assessment
      i. assess for Aura (sensation that warns of impending seizure)
      ii. Postictal state (period after seizure): memory loss, sleepiness, impaired speech
      iii. assess type, onset, duration
   b. Therapeutic Management
      i. Maintain patent airway
         1. turn client to side
         2. have O2 and suction equipment available after the seizure

             3. DO NOT force anything into the
                mouth during the seizure
                (including bite block)
       ii. prevent injury
             1. bed to the lowest position
             2. padded side rails
             3. loosen restrictive clothing
             4. DO NOT try to restrain client
       iii. Document onset, preceding events,
            duration, and postictal events
       iv. Medications
             1. Anitepileptics
             2. Diazepam, Lorazepam,
                phenobarbital are often given
                during seizure activity
       v. Educate client and family on importance
          of medication compliance
       vi. Educate family on care during seizure

Parkinson's Disease
   1. Overview
       a. Degenerative neurological disorder caused by
          atrophy of substantia negra leading to depletion
          of dopamine. This leads to termination of
          acetylcholine inhibition which causes symptoms.
       b. Dopamine plays a role in the inhibition of
          excitatory impulses. When this neurotransmitter is
          depleted acetylcholine is no longer inhibited.
       c. Slow, progressive disease.
       d. client becomes progressively debilitated and self-
          care dependent
   2. NCLEX® Points
       a. Assessment
           i. bradykinesia: slow movements due to
              muscle rigidity
           ii. resting tremor
           iii. Pill rolling - tremors in hands and fingers
           iv. Akinesia
           v. blank facial expression
           vi. shuffling steps, stooped stance, drooling

        vii. dysphagia
- b. Therapeutic Management
    - i. Assistive devices
    - ii. involvement of speech, physical, and occupational therapy
    - iii. monitor diet to insure proper caloric intake
        1. increase fluid intake
        2. high protein
        3. high fiber
    - iv. Assess ability to swallow prior to anything by mouth
    - v. Use rocking movement to initiate movement
    - vi. encourage client to ambulate multiple times a day
    - vii. participate in active and passive range of motion activities
    - viii. avoid foods high in Vitamin B6 (blocks effects of antiparkinsonian drugs)
    - ix. small, frequent, nutrient dense foods
    - x. Medication therapy
        1. dopaminergics, dopamine agonists, anticholinergics
        2. goal is to increase the level of dopamine in the CNS
        3. eventually drugs become ineffective

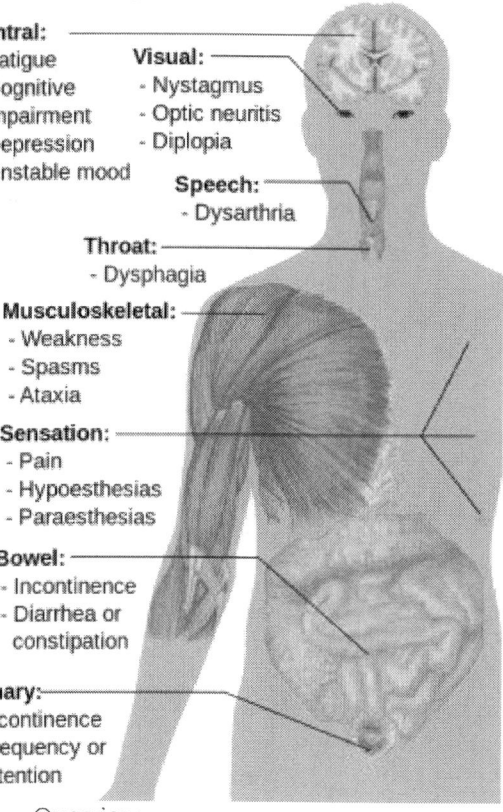

Main symptoms of
Multiple sclerosis

Central:
- Fatigue
- Cognitive impairment
- Depression
- Unstable mood

Visual:
- Nystagmus
- Optic neuritis
- Diplopia

Speech:
- Dysarthria

Throat:
- Dysphagia

Musculoskeletal:
- Weakness
- Spasms
- Ataxia

Sensation:
- Pain
- Hypoesthesias
- Paraesthesias

Bowel:
- Incontinence
- Diarrhea or constipation

Urinary:
- Incontinence
- Frequency or retention

1. Overview
   a. Chronic, progressive demyelinization of the neurons in the CNS
   b. Remission and exacerbation
   c. Primarily ages 20-40 years old
2. NCLEX® Points
   a. Assessment
      i. fatigue
      ii. tremors
      iii. spasticity of muscles
      iv. bladder dysfunction
      v. decrease peripheral sensation (pain, temperature, touch)

              vi. visual disturbances
             vii. emotional instability
      b. Therapeutic Management
             i. No cure - supportive therapy
             ii. energy conservation
             iii. maintain adequate fluid intake 2000 mL/day
             iv. provide bowel and bladder training
             v. encourage activity independence
             vi. regulate temperatures on water heaters, baths, and heating pads
             vii. insure in home safety (rugs, cords, etc)

Myasthenia Gravis

1. Overview
   a. Chronic progressive disorder of the PNS which affects transmission of nerve impulses
   b. Onset often caused by precipitating factors (stress, hormone disturbance, infection, trauma, temperature)
   c. Insufficient secretion of acetylcholine with excessive secretion of cholinesterase
2. NCLEX® Points
   a. Assessment
      i. weakness/fatigue
      ii. diplopia (double vision) and ptosis (drooping eyelid)

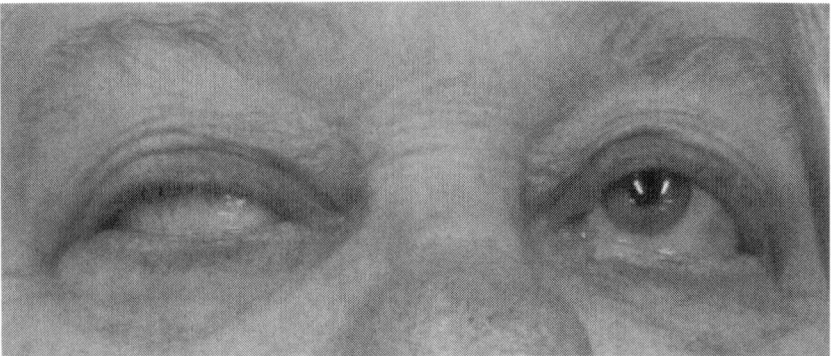

   iii. monitor respiratory status
- 1. swallowing, respirations, tachypnea, abnormal ABG, breath sounds, difficulty breathing

   iv. Cholinergic crisis: severe muscle weakness due to overmedication; cramps, diarrhea, bradycardia, bronchial spasm
- 1. Assessment
  - a. N/V, diarrhea
  - b. hypotension
  - c. blurred vision
- 2. Intervention
  - a. withhold medication
  - b. administer antidote

   v. Myasthenic crisis: acute exacerbation of disease, sudden severe motor weakness, risk of respiratory failure, caused by insufficient medication dosage
- 1. Assessment
  - a. increase pulse, respirations, bp
  - b. anoxia and cyanosis
  - c. bowel and bladder dysfunction
- 2. Intervention
  - a. increase medication

   vi. Tensilon test
- 1. used to confirm diagnosis
  - a. client at risk of vfib and cardiac arrest have atropine available

b. Therapeutic Management
   i. monitor respiratory status

ii. maintain suction and emergency equipment
iii. insure proper medication
iv. monitor feeding and insure proper nutrition
1. schedule medication 30-40 minutes prior to meals
v. provide adequate eye care
vi. instruct client to avoid temperature extremes, emotional stress, drugs, alcohol, and exposure to infection
vii. educate on signs of cholinergic and myasthenic crisis

NCLEX® Cram - Neurological Disorders
1. Glasgow Coma Scale

Score	1	2	3	4	5	6
Eyes	Does not open	Opens to painful stimuli	Opens to voice	Opens spontaneously	N/A	N/A
Verbal	Makes no sound	Incomprehensible sounds	Utters inappropriate words	Confused, disoriented	Oriented, converses normally	N/A
Motor	Makes no movements	Extension to painful stimuli	Flexion to painful stimuli	Withdraws to painful stimuli	Localizes to pain	Obeys commands

2. Hypothalamus
   a. regulates body temperature
   b. regulates response to sympathetic and parasympathetic nervous system
   c. produces hormones secreted by pituitary gland and hypothalamus
3. Pons
   a. regulates breathing
4. CT Scan

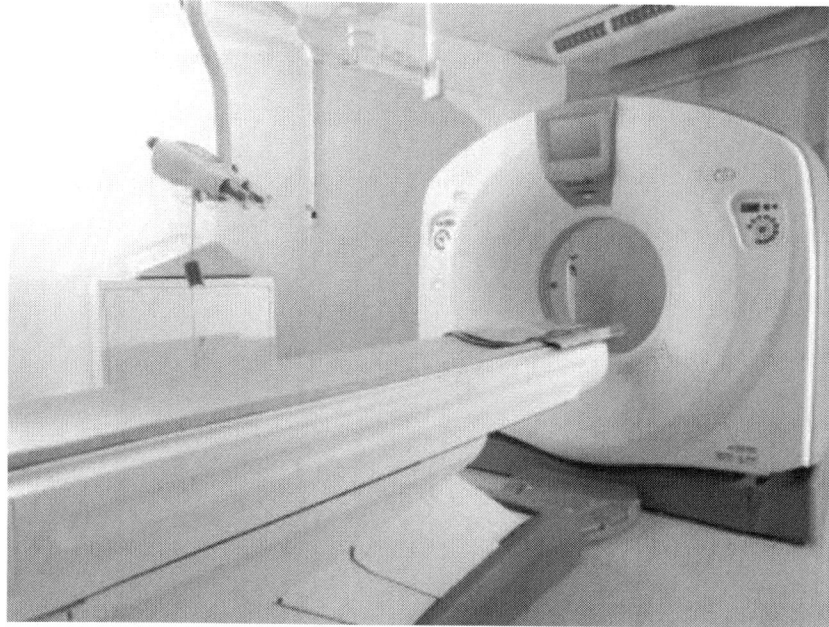

    a. assess for allergy to contrast, shellfish, iodine if dye is used

    b. provide adequate fluids to flush dye if used

5. MRI

    a. remove all metal objects from patients

    b. determine if client has a pacemaker - cannot complete MRI with pacemaker

6. Cerebral Angiography

    a. assess for allergies to dye

    b. maintain flat bed rest or at the position the physician orders

    c. assess insertion site for swelling, hematoma, and bleeding

7. Level of consciousness is the most essential indicator of neurological status

8. Pupil Assessment

    a. Pupils equal and react to light

    b. Pupil reacts slowly to light

    c. Dilated pupil (compressed cranial nerve III)

    d. Bilateral pupilary dilation, fixed (ominous)

    e. Bilateral pinpoint (pons damage)

9. Client position
    a. Decorticate
        i. flexes both arms on chest (toward CORd)
        ii. cortex damage

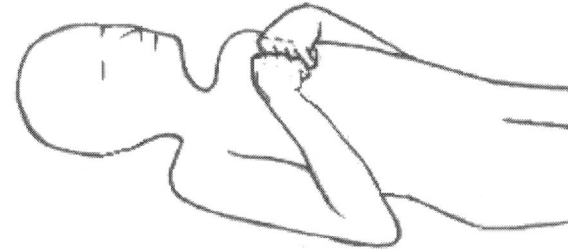

    b. Decerebrate
        i. extends arms and/or legs
        ii. brainstem lesion
    c. Flaccid
        i. no motor response to stimuli
10. Babinski test
    a. dorsiflexion of the big toe indicating neurologic damage

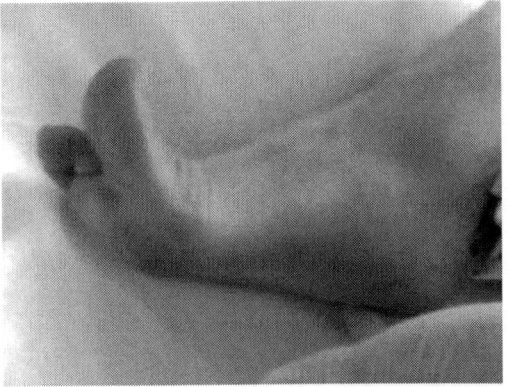

11. Hyperthermia can increase cerebral O2 demands and lead to hypoxia
    a. initiate seizure precautions
12. Halo Sign
    a. CSF will separate from blood when placed on a white sterile background

13. Do not suction or blow nose with traumatic head injury or pituitary surgery
14. Diabetes insipidus results from inadequate secretion of ADH and can be manifested as copious amounts of urine output. This reflects damage to the pituitary gland.
15. Immobilize clients when spinal injury is suspected
16. Clean pin sites on halo traction devices daily
    a. Do not shower
    b. keep pin sites clean, assess skin, report any redness or swelling
17. Turn spinal patients using the log rolling technique
18. Trigeminal Neuralgia
    a. damage to fifth cranial nerve
    b. severe pain to cheeks, lips, gums
    c. extreme temperatures may exacerbate symptoms
    d. client should avoid hot or cold foods and fluids
19. Bell's Palsy
    a. sudden weakness in the muscles on one half of face
    b. usually resolves within 6 months without treatment
    c. steroids and antivirals may be provided
    d. protect eyes from dryness
    e. chew food on unaffected side

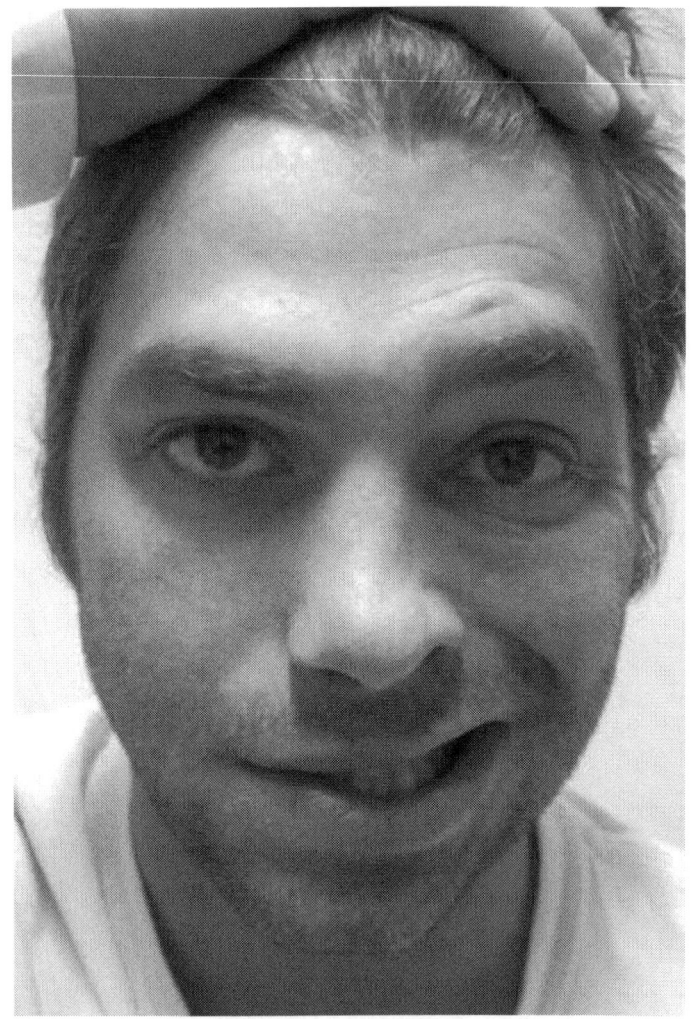

20. Guillain-Barre Syndrome
    a. monitor respiratory status closely
21. West Nile Virus
    a. symptoms develop 3-14 days after being bitten by infected mosquito

      b. fever, headache, tremors, seizures, coma, vision loss

      c. DEET bug spray should be worn

22. Meningitis

      a. inflammation of the brain and spinal cord membranes due to infection by virus, bacteria, or fungus, protozoa

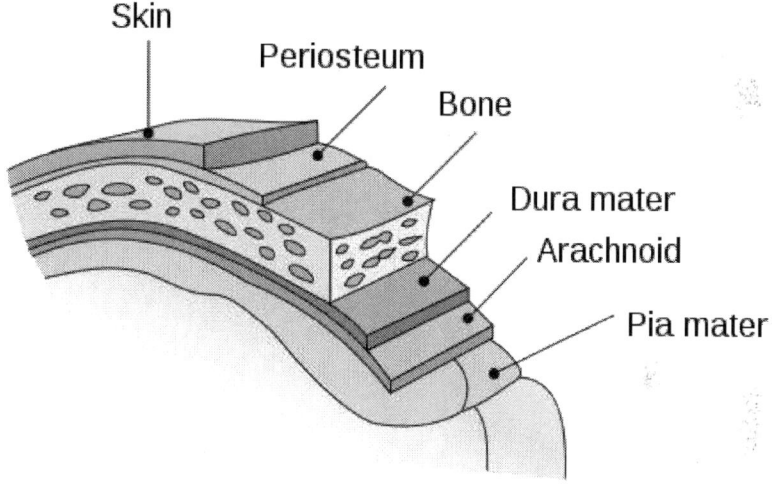

      b. CSF is analyzed to determine diagnosis

         i. cloudy, ↑WBC, ↓Glucose

      c. Nuchal rigidity

      d. photophobia

      e. lethargy

      f. altered level of consciousness

      g. positive Kernig and Burdzinski's sign

      h. client should be placed in isolation

      i. administer analgesics and antibiotics

      j. initiate seizure precautions

      k. Assess for ↑ICP

      l. Transmission usually occurs in areas of population density and crowded living spaces

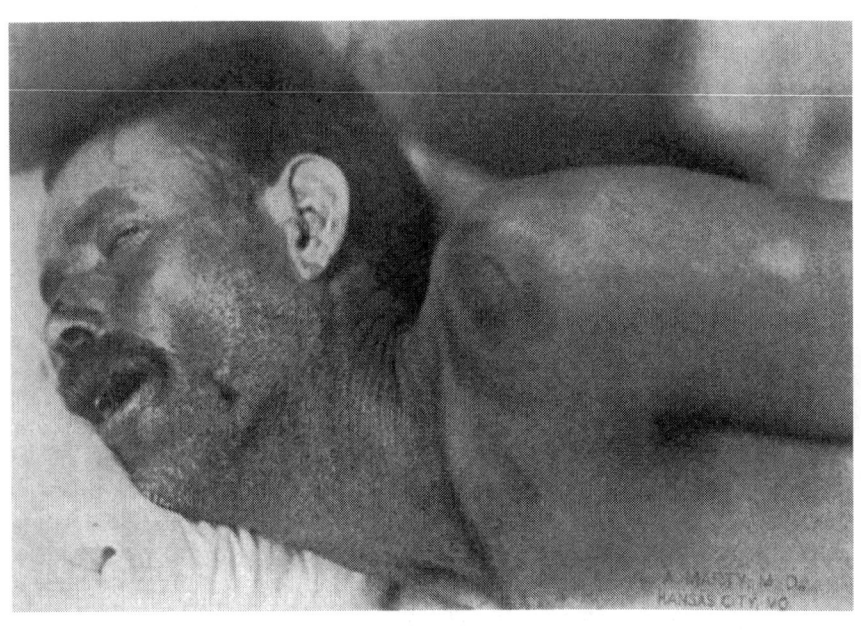

Acute Kidney Injury

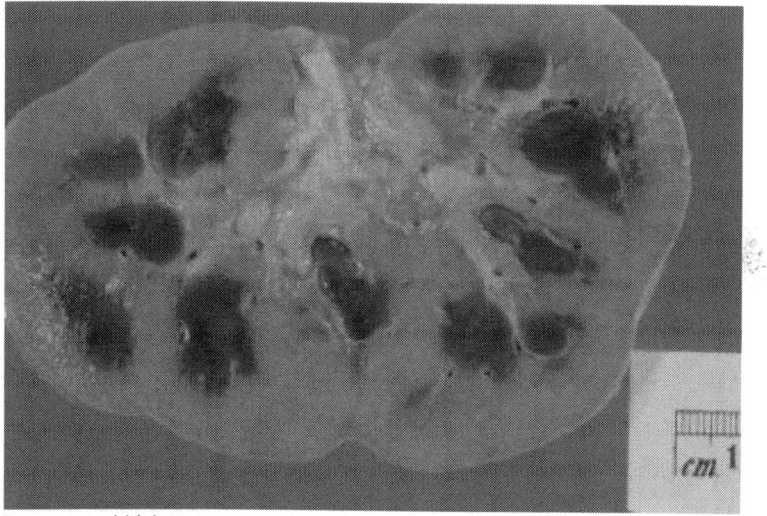

Damaged kidney

1. Overview
    a. Sudden loss of renal function due to poor circulation or renal cell damage
    b. usually reversible may resolve on its own, can lead to permanent damage if not reversed quickly
    c. Causes
        i. Prerenal: decreased blood flow to kidneys, accounts for majority of cases
        ii. Intrarenal: within the kidney due to tubular necrosis, infection, obstruction, prolonged ischemia
        iii. Postrenal: damage between the kidney and urethral meatus generally caused by infection, calculi, obstruction
    d. Phases
        i. Progresses in phases
            1. Onset
            2. Oliguric
                a. decreased urine output <400 mL/day

                    b. signs of hypervolemia
                       (HTN, HF, edema,
                       pericardial effusion)
                    c. pericarditis
                    d. Therapeutic
                       Management
                            i. restrict fluid
                               intake
                            ii. identify cause
                            iii. diuretics
          3. Diuretic
                    a. gradual urine output
                       increase followed by
                       diuresis
                    b. Therapeutic
                       Management
                            i. replace fluids
                               and electrolytes
          4. Recovery
          ii. Can progress to chronic kidney injury if
              not reversed
          iii. Signs and symptoms result from kidneys
               inability to regulate fluid and electrolytes
2. NCLEX® Points
     a. Assessment
          i. Azotemia (retention of nitrogen waste in
             blood)
          ii. monitor urine output
          iii. monitor weight daily
          iv. monitor for infection
          v. monitor for fluid overload (edema,
             crackles, wheezes)
          vi. monitor for metabolic acidosis
          vii. prepare for dialysis

Chronic Kidney Disease
1. Overview
     a. Progressive, irreversible loss of renal function with
        associated decline in GFR
     b. all body systems affected dialysis is required

      c. ESRD occurs with GFR <15mL/min

      d. Causes

          i. DM

          ii. HTN

          iii. unreversed AKI

          iv. glomerulonephritis

          v. autoimmune disorders

2. NCLEX® Points

    a. Assessment

        i. azotemia

        ii. ↑BUN, creatinine

        iii. Cardio

           1. HTN, hypervolemia, CHF

        iv. Hematologic

           1. anemia

           2. thrombocytopenia

        v. Gastrointestinal

           1. anorexia

           2. N/V

        vi. Neurological

           1. lethargy

           2. confusion

           3. coma

        vii. Urinary

           1. ↓ urine output

           2. proteinuria

        viii. Skeletal

           1. osteoporosis

    b. Therapeutic Management

        i. epoetin alfa aids in countering anemia

        ii. avoid administering asprin

        iii. monitor potassium levles

           1. ↑ potassium can lead to EKG changes (peaked T waves, flat P, wide QRS, blocks, asystole)

           2. provide low potassium diet

           3. Potassium lowering medications

               a. Kayexalate

               b. insulin

        c. calcium gluconate

     4. provide continuous cardiac monitoring

iv. phosphate binders may be required to lower phosphorus levels

v. monitor daily weights

vi. monitor for signs of heart failure

vii. monitor electrolyte levels and BUN Creatinine

viii. assess peripheral nerve function and monitor for peripheral neuropathy

ix. vision can be affected: monitor and provide for a safe environment

x. instruct client on dialysis and provide end of life care as needed

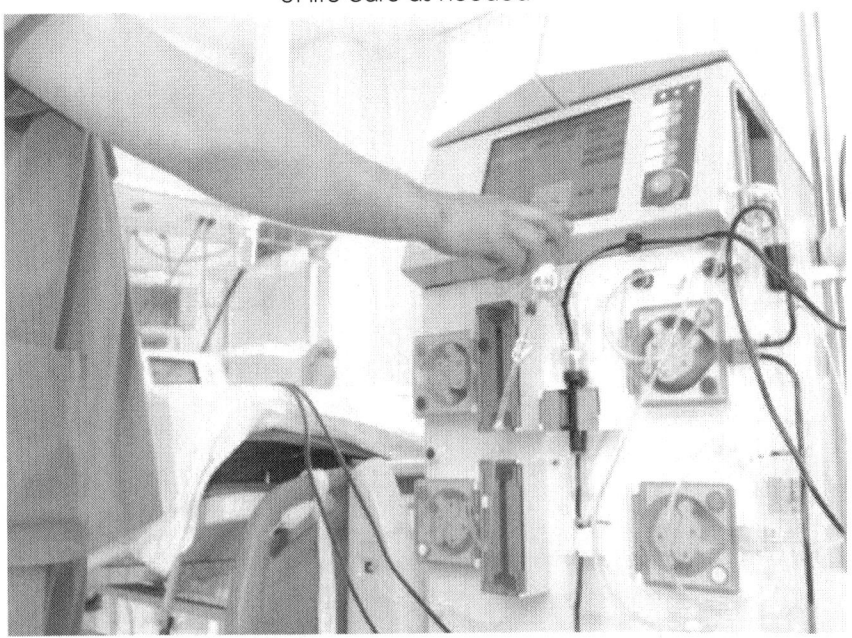

Renal Calculi

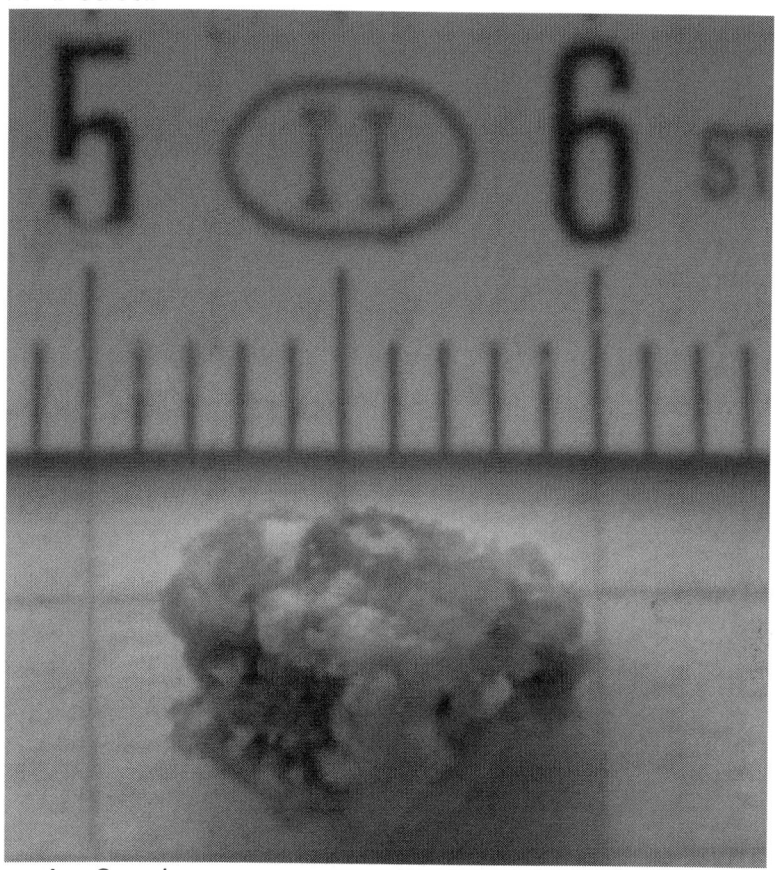

1. Overview
   a. Stones that form in the urinary tract
   b. Form as a result of chemicals in urine becoming concentrated (calcium or oxalate, struvite, uric acid, cystine)
   c. Causes
      i. diet high in calcium, Vit D, protein, purines
      ii. dehydration
      iii. immobilization
      iv. ↑uric acid (gout)
      v. infection
      vi. obstruction

2. NCLEX® Points
   a. Assessment
      i. pain which radiates from lumbar to side to testicles or bladder
      ii. severe pain with sudden onset
      iii. dull pain in renal area
      iv. signs of UTI
      v. hematuria (blood in urine)
   b. Therapeutic Management
      i. monitor VS looking for infection
      ii. increase fluid intake to 3000 mL/day
      iii. provide analgesia to treat pain
      iv. promote ambulation
      v. strain all urine to catch stone
      vi. Treatment options
         1. Extracoporeal Shock-wave Lithotripsy (ESWL)
            a. external shock waves generated to pulverize stone
         2. Lithotomy
            a. surgical removal
         3. Nephrostomy
            a. small flank incision with stone removal via endoscope
         4. Uroscopy
            a. urethral catheter inserted via cystoscope

Glomerulonephritis
1. Overview
   a. Inflammatory disorder of the glomerulus caused by immunological reaction
   b. Predisposing factors
      i. upper respiratory infection
      ii. skin infection
      iii. SLE
2. NCLEX® Points
   a. Assessment

      i.   fever
     ii.   anorexia, N/V
    iii.   malaise
    iv. ↑BUN and Creatinine, ↓Creatinine clearance
     v. ↓ uptake and excretion of dye with renal scan
    vi. HTN
   vii. Hypoalbuminemia
  viii. hematuria, protneinuria
b. Therapeutic Management
      i.   Plasmapheresis: removal of harmful antibodies from plasma
     ii.   dialysis
    iii.   protein restriction, ↓K+, ↓Na+
    iv. bedrest
     v. monitor daily weight and I&O

Nephrotic Syndrome

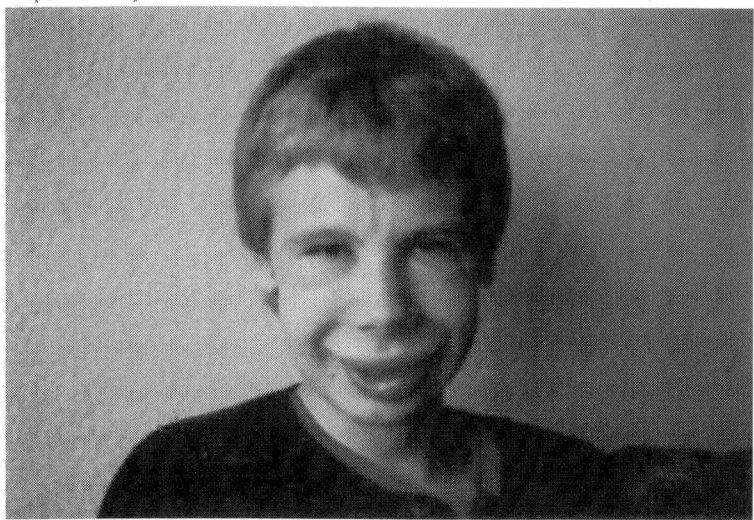

Facial edema from sodium and water retention caused by nephrotic syndrome

1. Overview
   a. Kidney disease characterized by loss of protein from plasma into urine
   b. proteinurea, hypoalbuminemia, edema

        c.   Plasma proteins leak into the urine, fluid shift occurs leading to massive edema

2.   NCLEX® Points

    a.   Assessment

        i.   severe edema

        ii.   weight gain

        iii.   renal failure symptoms

        iv.   fatigue

        v.   amenorrhea

        vi.   positive renal biopsy

    b.   Therapeutic Management

        i.   goal is to reduce urinary protein excretion, reduce edema, minimize further complications

        ii.   ↓Na in diet

        iii.   high protein diet

        iv.   bed rest

        v.   monitor immunologic function

           1.   assess for infection

           2.   Monitor CBC with attention on WBC and differential

           3.   hand hygiene

Urinary Tract Infection (UTI)
1. Overview
   a. infection within the urinary tract leading to inflammation
   b. urinary tract is sterile above the urethra, pathogens gain entrance via perineal area or via bloodstream
   c. females are more prone due to shorter urethra
   d. males become more susceptible with age due to urinary stasis
2. NCLEX® Points
   a. Assessment
      i. Urine
         1. cloudy, frequent, strong odor, burning, frequent
      ii. **Confusion (altered mental status) and lethargy in older adults**
      iii. ↑WBCs
      iv. urine cultures reveal bacteria
   b. Therapeutic Management
      i. ↑fluid intake (3000 mL/day)
      ii. antimicrobials
      iii. urine cultures
      iv. antimicrobials, antispasmodics, analgesics
      v. Client education
         1. avoid caffeine, carbonation, alcohol
         2. complete the course of antibiotics
         3. ↑fluid intake
         4. avoid powder, sprays, avoid baths
         5. frequent urination
         6. drink cranberry juice

Benign Prostatic Hyperplasia (BPH)

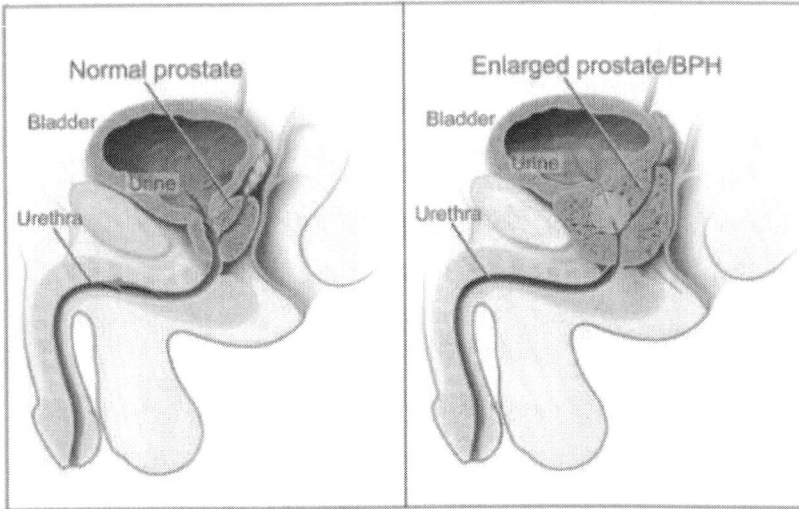

1. Overview
    a. enlargement of the prostate gland leading to
       partial or total obstruction of the urethra
2. NCLEX® Points
    a. Assessment
        i. feeling of incomplete bladder emptying
        ii. ↓force of urine stream
        iii. nocturia
        iv. postvoid dribbling
        v. urinary stasis
        vi. UTIs
        vii. hematuria
    b. Therapeutic Management
        i. ↑ fluid intake (3000mL/day)
        ii. avoid anything that leads to urinary
            retention
        iii. follow medication regimen
        iv. create and follow voiding schedule
        v. ↓caffeine, artificial sweeteners, spicy and
            acidic foods
        vi. TURP - transurethral resection of the
            prostate

1. Hemodialysis
   a. process of cleaning the blood of waste and toxins by diffusion across a semipermeable membrane
   b. cleanses the clients blood
   c. removes urea, creatinine, uric acid
   d. monitor vital signs closely throughout
   e. monitor labs values closely
   f. weigh the client before and after dialysis to estimate fluid loss
   g. assess for bleeding
   h. hold antihypertensives and medications that might affect blood pressure
   i. hold medications that will be removed by dialysis (contact pharmacy with questions)
   j. Do not use hemodialysis access catheters for anything other than hemodialysis
   k. do not insert IVs on extremity with active shunt
   l. do not assess blood pressure on affected extremity
   m. assess capillary refill in affected extremity
   n. monitor fistulas and grafts closely for clots
      i. Bruit: listen
      ii. Thrill: feel
      iii. Always assess for a bruit and thrill with ESRD patients. If bruit and thrill are absent notify the physician.
   o. complication with dialysis are severe (air embolus, electrolyte imbalance, shock, hemorrhage, sepsis, encephalopathy)
      i. monitor and assess the client thoroughly and frequently
2. Peritoneal Dialysis

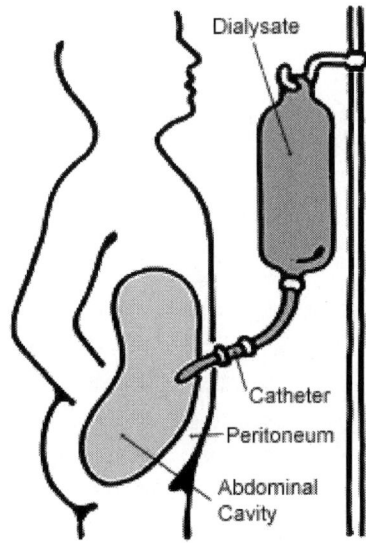

Dialysate

Catheter

Peritoneum

Abdominal Cavity

    a. peritoneum acts as semipermeable membrane
        i. contraindications
            1. peritonitis
            2. abdominal surgery
        ii. can be continuous (24/7)
    b. complications
        i. peritonitis (infection of the peritoneum)
        ii. cloudy outflow sign of peritonitis and should be reported
        iii. avoid infection via strict sterile technique

3. Function of the kidneys
    a. maintain acid-base balance
    b. fluid and electrolyte balance
    c. secrete renin to aid in blood pressure regulation and erythropoietin (stimulate bone marrow to produce RBCs)
    d. urine production

4. Creatinine clearance used to estimate GFR (normal 125 mL/minute, decreases with age)

5. Assess allergy to dye, shellfish, iodine prior to urography
    a. instruct to drink fluids to flush dye post procedure unless contraindicated
    b. dye damaging to kidneys

6. Cystoscopy used to examine bladder and take biopsy: https://youtu.be/d9Vx3Lgz4sw
7. Renal biopsy
    a. assess coagulation studies
    b. assess client for bleeding from site post procedure
    c. apply pressure to site
8. Urosepsis
    a. most common cause is a urinary catheter
9. Hydronephrosis
    a. renal distention caused by obstruction of normal urine flow
        i. monitor fluid and electrolyte balance

Gastrointestinal Disorders

Gastroesophageal Reflux Disease (GERD)

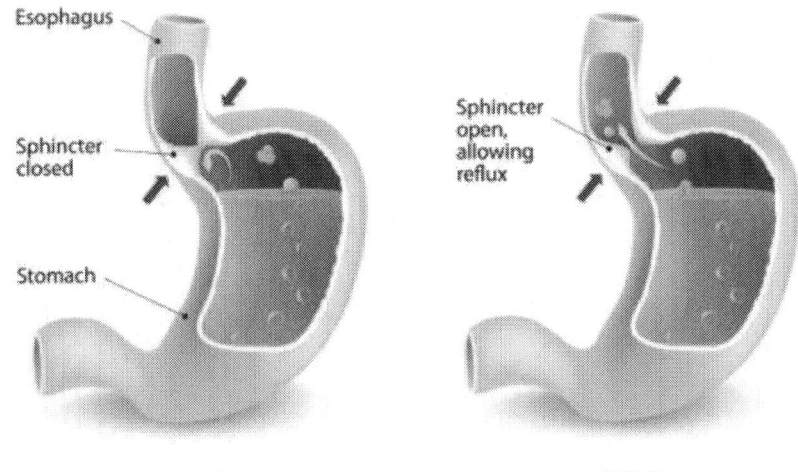

Healthy   **GERD**

1. Overview
    a. Backward movement of gastric contents into esophagus
    b. Due to relaxation of or incompetent lower esophageal sphincter, pyloric stenosis, increased gastric volume, or motility disorder
2. NCLEX® Points
    a. Assessment
        i. heartburn
            1. exacerbated by bending over, straining, or recumbent position
        ii. regurgitation
        iii. hypersalivation
        iv. difficulty swallowing
        v. dyspepsia (discomfort in upper abdomen)
    b. Therapeutic Management
        i. Diagnosis made via pH test, esophagoscopy used to rule out malignancy

        ii.   do not eat within 2 hours of bedtime

        iii. avoid food that reduce lower esophageal sphincter tone

            1. peppermint

            2. chocolate

            3. carbonated beverages

            4. smoking

            5. fried and fatty foods

        iv. eat a low fat, high fiber diet

        v.   avoid medications that ↓ gastric emptying (anticholinergics)

        vi. elevate HOB while sleeping

        vii. Medications

            1. antiacids

            2. H2 receptor antagonists

            3. Proton pump inhibitors

Peptic Ulcer Disease

1. Overview
   a. Break in mucosal lining of stomach, pylorus, duodenum, or esophagus that come in contact with gastric secretions
2. NCLEX® Points
   a. Assessment
      i. pain
         1. Gastric
            a. gnawing, sharp 30-60 after a meal
         2. Duodenal
            a. 1.5 to 3 hours after eating
            b. relieved by eating
      ii. Upper GI series and EGD used to diagnose
      iii. hematemesis (gastric)
      iv. melena (duodenal)
   b. Therapeutic Management
      i. avoid foods that cause irritation
         1. coffee
         2. cola

            3. tea
            4. chocolate
            5. high sodium
            6. spicy foods
        ii. smoking cessation
        iii. small, frequent meals
        iv. avoid aspirin and NSAIDs
        v. monitor H&H and assess for bleeding
        vi. Surgical options
            1. gastrectomy
            2. vagotomy
            3. gastric resection
            4. Bilroth I, Bilroth II
        vii. medications
            1. H2 receptor antagonists
            2. Proton pump inhibitors
            3. Antacids
            4. sucralfate (Carafate)

Hiatal Hernia

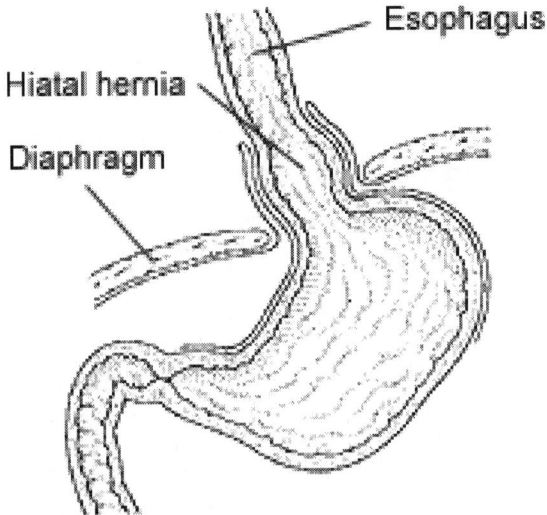

1. Overview
    a. Protrusion of bowel through the diaphragm into thorax

        b.   due to weakening of muscles in diaphragm
2. NCLEX® Points
    a.   Assessment
        i.   heartburn
        ii.   regurgitation
        iii.   dysphagia
        iv.   fullness
        v.   bowel sounds over chest
    b.   Therapeutic Management
        i.   similar to GERD
        ii.   do not lay down for 1 hour after eating
        iii.   avoid medications that delay gastric emptying (anticholinergics)
        iv.   eat small, frequent meals
        v.   avoid straining
        vi.   avoid vigorous exercise
        vii.   sleep with HOB elevated

Inflammatory Bowel Disease (IBD)

Ulcerative Colitis
1. Overview
    a.   chronic inflammation of mucosa and submucosa in colon and rectum
    b.   results in poor absorption of nutrients
    c.   progresses upward from rectum to cecum
    d.   perforation may develop as colon becomes edematous leading to lesions and ulcers
    e.   exacerbation and remission episodes
2. NCLEX® Points
    a.   Assessment
        i.   10-20 liquid stools per day containing blood and mucus
        ii.   malnutrition, dehydration, electrolyte imbalances
        iii.   anorexia
    b.   Therapeutic Management
        i.   Maintain NPO during acute phase administering IV fluids and electrolytes
        ii.   reduce intestinal activity

      iii. assess stool
              1. assess for blood
      iv. monitor for bowel perforation and hemorrhage
      v. diet therapy
              1. low residue
              2. high protein
              3. high calorie
              4. vitamins and iron
      vi. avoid foods that may exacerbate symptoms
              1. raw vegetables and fruits
              2. nuts
              3. popcorn
              4. whole-grain
              5. cereals
              6. spicy
      vii. medications
              1. corticosteroids
              2. salicylates
              3. immunomodulators
              4. antidirrheals

Crohn's Disease

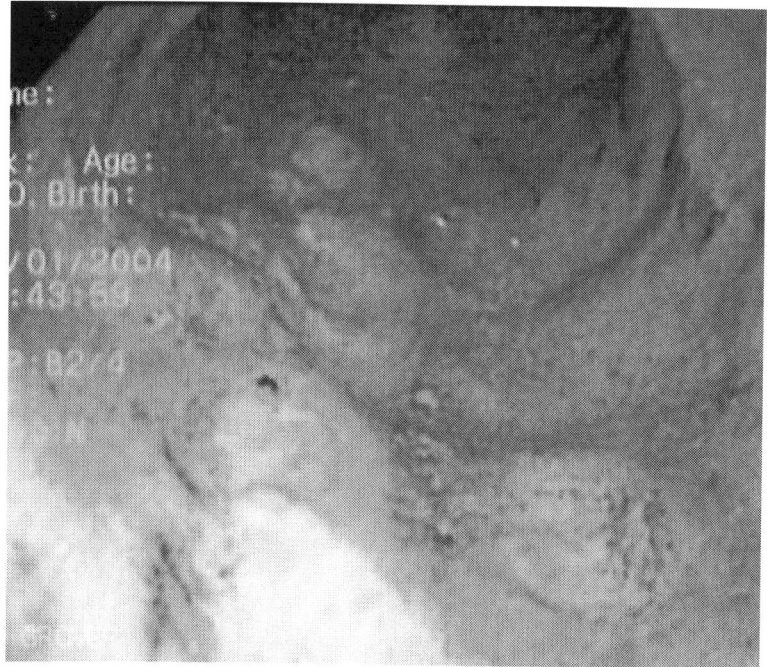

1. Overview
    a. inflammatory disease of GI mucosa anywhere from mouth to anus most often affecting the terminal ileum
    b. leads to thickening and scarring, ulcerations and abscesses
    c. remissions and exacerbations
2. NCLEX® Points
    a. Assessment
        i. fever
        ii. cramps and pain after meals (relieved by defecation)
        iii. diarrhea containing mucus or pus (5-6 stools/day)
        iv. anemia

    v. electrolyte imbalances
    vi. malnutrition
   b. Therapeutic Management
    i. diet
     1. high calorie
     2. high protein
    ii. medications - similar to ulcerative colitis
    iii. weigh daily and maintain accurate I&O

Appendicitis

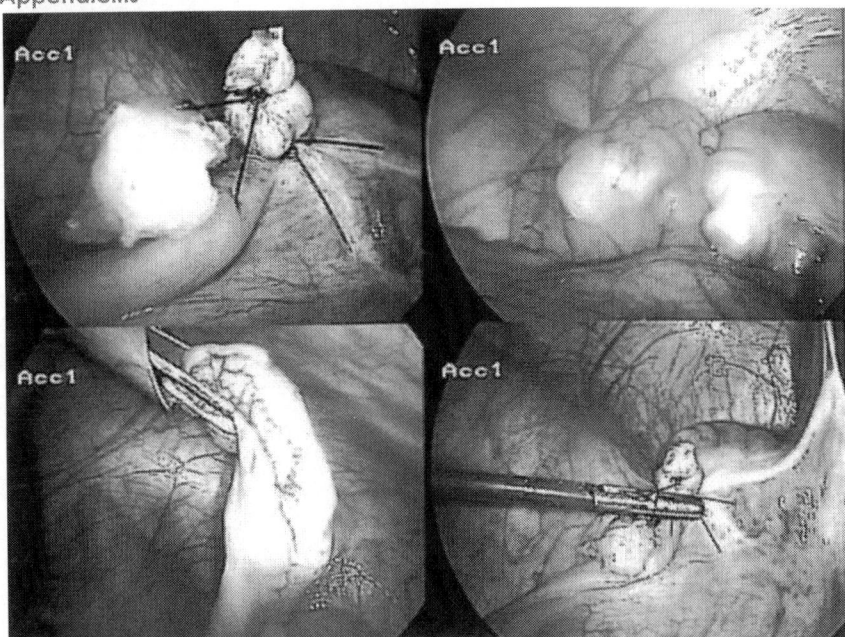

1. Overview
  a. Inflammation of the appendix
  b. major risk factor is appendix rupture leading to peritonitis and/or sepsis
2. NCLEX® Points
  a. Assessment
    i. abdominal pain at McBurney's point
    ii. pain descends to RLQ
    iii. ↑WBC
    iv. rebound tenderness
    v. fever

<pre>
                    vi. abdominal guarding
                    vii. sudden relief of pain indicates rupture
            b. Therapeutic Management
                    i. Appendectomy
                            1. keep client NPO
                            2. avoid heat application which
                                can lead to rupture
                            3. avoid stimulation of peristalsis
                            4. if rupture occurs, postoperative
                                healing is prolonged will have
                                drains and NG tube for
                                decompression
                            5. monitor VS and assess for
                                abdominal distention post
                                operatively
</pre>

Diverticulitis and Diverticulosis

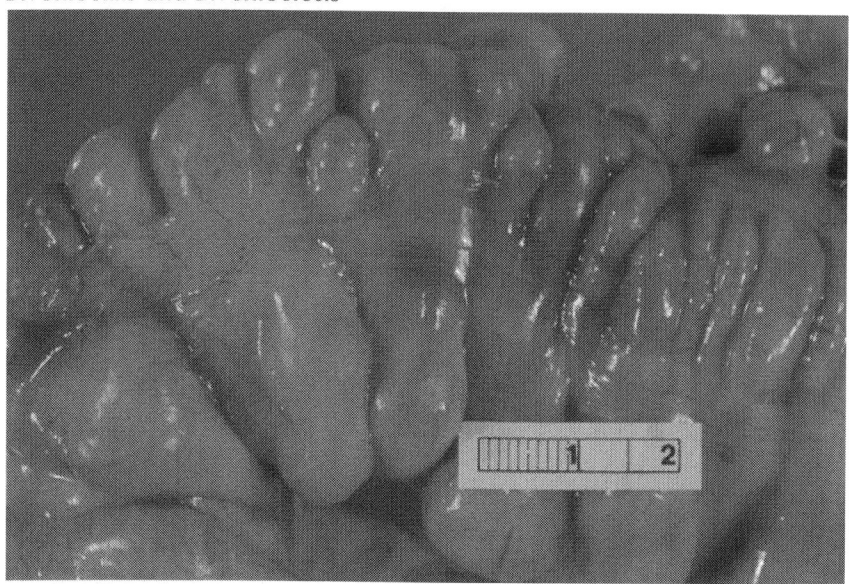

1. Overview
    a. Diverticulosis
        i. Outpouching of intestinal mucosa
    b. Diverticulitis
        i. Inflammation of one or more
           diverticulosis due to trapped food or

bacteria can lead to perforation and peritonitis

2. NCLEX® Points
    a. Assessment
        i. LLQ pain worsening with straining
        ii. ↑temp
        iii. N/V
        iv. Abdominal distention
        v. Melena
    b. Therapeutic Management
        i. NPO - bowel rest
        ii. bedrest
        iii. introduce fiber slowly
        iv. ↑ fluid intake
        v. avoid gas forming foods
        vi. bulk forming laxatives
        vii. avoid nuts, foods with small seeds

Hemorrhoids

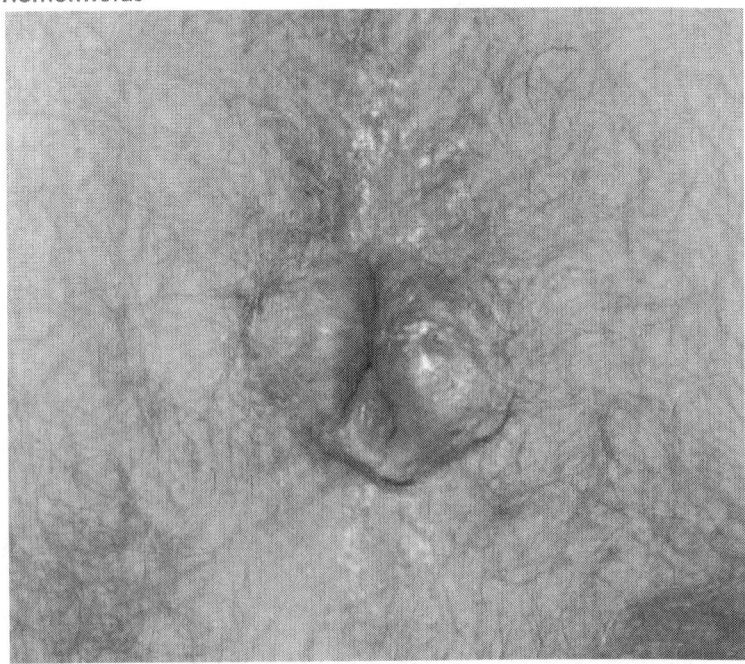

1. Overview

        a. swollen and inflamed veins of the anus and lower rectum

        b. caused by straining, portal hypertension, irritation

        c. internal, external, or prolapsed

2. NCLEX® Points

        a. Assessment

            i. rectal pain

           ii. bright red bleeding with defecation

        b. Therapeutic Management

            i. sitz-bath

           ii. high fiber diet

          iii. ↑ fluid intake

          iv. stool softeners

           v. cold packs and analgesics

Cholecystitis
1. Overview
    a. acute or chronic inflammation of the gall bladder most often caused by gall stones (cholelithiasis)
2. NCLEX® Points
    a. Assessment
        i. N/V
        ii. RUQ pain
            1. can occur 2-4 hours after high fat meals
            2. lasting 1-3 hours
        iii. Murphy's Sign
            1. pain with expiration while examiners hand is placed below the costal margin on right side at midclavicular line. Patient then asked to inspire if patient is unable to inspire due to pain, test is positive.
        iv. rebound tenderness
    b. Therapeutic Management
        i. NPO
        ii. antiemetics
        iii. nasogastric decompression
        iv. analgesics
        v. avoid gas forming foods
        vi. surgery
            1. cholecystectomy
                a. removal of gall bladder
                b. monitor for pain and infection at incision site
                c. abdominal splinting when coughing
                d. T-tube
                    i. High Fowlers position
                        1. report drainag

e
>500mL

Hepatitis
1. Overview
    a. inflammation of liver
    b. severity varies from mild cases with liver cell regeneration to severe cases with hepatic necrosis and cell death within weeks
    c. Forms
        i. Hepatitis A (HAV)
            1. health care workers at risk
            2. Transmission
                a. fecal-oral
                b. person-to-person
                c. poorly washed hands/utensils
                d. contagious
                    i. most contagious 10-14 days prior to onset of symptoms
                e. self limiting
            3. Prevention
                a. strict hand washing best preventative measure
                b. Hepatitis A vaccine
        ii. Hepatitis B (HBV)
            1. health care workers at risk
            2. Transmission
                a. IV drugs
                b. blood or body fluids
                c. sexual contact
            3. Prevention
                a. hand washing
                b. blood screening
                c. Hepatitis B vaccine
                d. needle precautions
                e. safe sex practices

iii. Hepatitis C (HCV)
  1. health care workers at risk
  2. Transmission
     a. IV drug users
     b. blood
  3. Prevention
     a. hand hygiene
     b. needle safety
     c. blood screening
iv. Hepatitis D (HDV)
v. Hepatitis E (HEV)

2. NCLEX® Points
   a. Assessment
      i. Preicteric Stage
         1. flulike symptoms
         2. pain
         3. low grade fever
      ii. Icteric Stage
         1. jaundice
         2. ↑bilirubin
         3. dark urine
         4. clay colored stool
      iii. Posticteric Stage
         1. recovery phase
         2. laboratory values return to normal
         3. pain relief
         4. increased energy
      iv. Laboratory values
         1. ↑ALT, AST, Ammonia, Billirubin

Cirrhosis

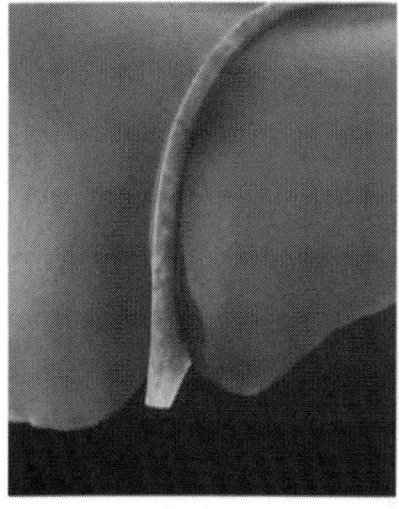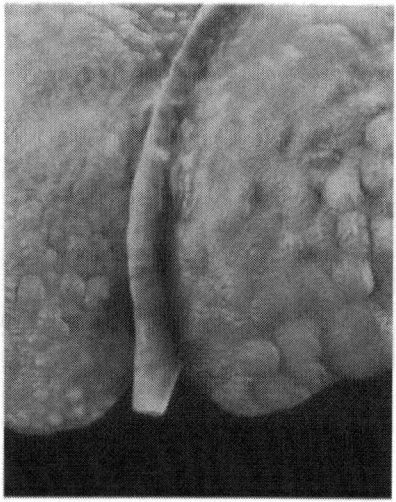

healthy   cirrhosis

1. Overview
   a. chronic, irreversible liver disease
   b. inflammation and fibrosis of liver cells
      (hepatocytes) leads to formation of scar tissue
      within liver which causes obstruction of hepatic
      blood flow and impedes proper liver function
         i. interruption of blood flow causes
            1. edema
            2. ascites
            3. esophageal varices
            4. hemorrhoids
            5. varicose veins

2. NCLEX® Points
    a. Assessment
        i. malaise
        ii. jaundice with scleral icterus
        iii. edema
        iv. anorexia
        v. clay-colored stool
        vi. pain in RUQ
        vii. hepatomegaly
        viii. splenomegaly
        ix. ascites (positive fluid wave test)
        x. hepatic encephalopathy
            1. disorientation
            2. altered LOC
            3. fatigue
        xi. asterixis (flapping hand tremor)
        xii. ↓reflexes
        xiii. anemia
        xiv. dark urine
    b. Complications
        i. portal hypertension
            1. increased pressure in portal vein
        ii. ascites
            1. fluid accumulation in abdominal cavity
        iii. esophageal varices
            1. dilated, thin veins in the esophagus can rupture
            2. bleeding is an life-threatening emergency
            3. goal is to control bleeding
        iv. Hepatorenal syndrome
            1. renal failure associated with liver failure
    c. Therapeutic Management
        i. elevate HOB
        ii. parecentesis to drain abdominal fluid
        iii. fluid restriction
        iv. ↓protein intake

v. ↓ Na intake
vi. monitor daily weights
vii. institute bleeding precautions and monitor coagulation studies
viii. Medications
1. vitamin K
2. antacids
3. lactulose to decrease ammonia levels
4. analgesics
5. blood products
6. diuretics

Pancreatitis

1. Overview
   a. inflammation of the pancreas
   b. autodigestion of pancreas results
   c. Alcohol abuse, gall bladder disease, PUD, obstruction of the ducts and hyperlipidemia common causes
   d. Acute - occurs suddenly with most patients recovering fully
   e. Chronic - usually due to longstanding alcohol abuse with loss of pancreatic function
2. NCLEX® Points
   a. abdominal pain
      i. sudden onset
      ii. mid epigastric
      iii. LUQ
   b. N/V
   c. weight loss
   d. abdominal tenderness
   e. ↑WBC, bilirubin, ALP, amylase, lipase
   f. Cullen's sign
      i. bruising and edema around the umbilicus
   g. Turner's sign
      i. flank bruising
   h. steatorrhea
3. Therapeutic Management

a. ↓pancreatic secretions
b. NPO
c. NG tube insertion to decompress stomach and suppress pancreatic secretions
d. IV hydration
e. TPN for prolonged exacerbations
f. educate on avoidance of alcohol
g. notify provider of exacerbations
h. ERCP to remove gall stones
i. medications
    i. analgesics
    ii. H2 blockers
    iii. Proton pump inhibitors
    iv. insulin
    v. anticholinergics

NCLEX® Cram - Gastrointestinal Disorders

1. Functions of the liver
    a. store vitamin B112 and fat-soluble vitamins
    b. store and release blood
    c. produce plasma proteins
    d. synthesize clotting factors
    e. convert amino acids to carbohydrates
    f. synthesize glucose
    g. detoxify alcohol and drugs
2. Functions of the pancreas
    a. secrete insulin and glucagon
    b. secrete sodium bicarbonate
    c. secrete pancreatic enzymes (amylase, lipase)
3. EGD
    a. keep client NPO for 6-12 hours prior
    b. keep client NPO until gag reflex returns
4. Colonoscopy

COLONOSCOPY

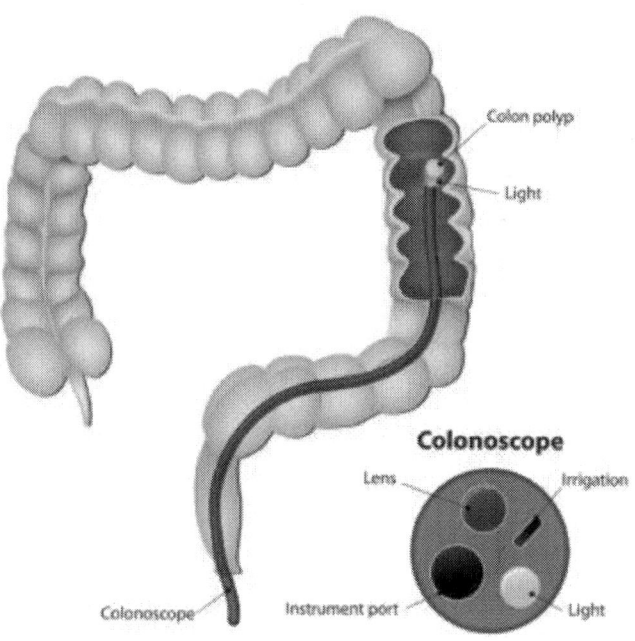

a. position
   i. side lying (left side) knees drawn up to chest
b. colon must be clean prior to procedure

5. Paracentesis
    a. removal of fluid from the peritoneal cavity
        i. monitor vital signs closely
        ii. monitor breathing - rapid fluid removal can lead to shock
        iii. Position
            1. upright, back supported
        iv. measure fluid collected
6. Liver biopsy
    a. monitor for bleeding
        i. high risk for bleeding
    b. position post procedure
        i. right side
        ii. pillow under costal margin
7. GI Surgery
    a. Colonostomy
        i. low-residue (low fiber) diet
        ii. assess appearance of stoma
            1. notify provider if stoma becomes pale, darkened, cyanotic, or bleeding increases
        iii. insure proper fit of pouch
            1. 1/8 inch between stoma and bag
            2. empty bag when 1/3 full
8. Pernicious anemia
    a. body unable to absorb vitamin B12
    b. requires monthly B12 injections
9. Dumping syndrome
    a. complication of gastric surgery (common with Billroth I and II)
        i. rapid emptying of gastric contents into small intestine without proper digestion
        ii. symptoms begin 30 minutes after eating
        iii. N/V
        iv. abdominal fullness
        v. palpitations
        vi. tachycardia
10. BMI

a. BMI = wt (kg)/Ht^2(m)
11. Malnutrition
    a. signs
        i. dry skin
        ii. anemia
        iii. muscle wasting
        iv. alopecia
        v. cheilosis (dry scaling lips)
        vi. glossitis
12. Melena - bloody stool
13. Steatorrhea - fat in stool
14. Intestinal obstruction
    a. assessment
        i. early - high pitched bowel sounds
        ii. late - absent
        iii. vomit with fecal scent
        iv. abdominal distention
    b. maintain NPO
15. Jaundice
    a. due to hyperbilirunemia
        i. bilirubin is a byproduct of hemoglobin breakdown
        ii. with liver damage bilirubin is not broken down
16. Ammonia
    a. byproduct of protein digestion in large intestine
    b. protein -> ammonia -> urea -> excreted via urine
    c. liver converts ammonia to urea
        i. with liver damage - ammonia levels raise in blood - causing complications and neurologic changes
        ii. lactulose draws ammonia from the blood into the urine to be excreted via stool
    d. BUN - measure renal and liver function
        i. ↑BUN = kidneys are not able to excrete urea
        ii. ↓BUN = liver is not converting ammonia to urea

17. Liver cancer
    a. RUQ pain, fatigue, anorexia, ascites, jaundice, liver failure
18. Pancreatic cancer
    a. causes
        i. smoking
        ii. toxins
        iii. high fat diet
    b. slow onset
    c. most clients do not present with symptoms until disease is advanced
    d. supportive care
    e. symptoms
        i. pain - worse when lying down
        ii. jaundice
        iii. weight loss
        iv. steatorrhea
19. Celiac Disease
    a. gluten sensitivity
    b. lifelong dietary modifications required
    c. Celiac Crisis
        i. acute episode
            1. precipitated by infection
            2. fasting
            3. gluten ingestion
            4. leads to: dehydration, electrolyte imbalance, severe acidosis
        ii. Assessment
            1. severe steatorrhea
            2. abdominal distention
            3. anemia
        iii. instruct patient on reading food labels

Metabolic and Endocrine Disorders

Syndrome of Inappropriate Antidiuretic Hormone (SIADH)
1. Overview
    a. Excess secretion of ADH from posterior pituitary leading to hyponatremia and water intoxication
    b. caused by trauma, tumors, infection, medications
2. NCLEX® Points
    a. Assessment
        i. fluid volume excess
            1. ↑BP
            2. crackles
            3. JVD
        ii. altered LOC
        iii. seizures
        iv. coma
        v. urine specific gravity >1.032
        vi. ↓BUN, hematocrit, Na+
    b. Therapeutic Management
        i. cardiac monitoring
        ii. frequent neurological examination
        iii. monitor I&O
        iv. fluid restriction
        v. Na supplement
        vi. daily weight (loss of 2.2 lbs or 1kg = about 1L)
        vii. Medication
            1. hypertonic saline
            2. diuretics
            3. electrolyte replacement

Diabetes Insipidus
1. Overview
    a. hyposecretion or failure to respond to ADH from posterior pituitary leading to excess water loss
    b. urine output ranging from 4L to 30L in a 24 hour period leads to dehydration
    c. Causes

           i. neurogenic, stroke, tumor, infection, pituitary surgery

2. NCLEX® Points
   a. Assessment
      i. excessive urine output
         1. dilute urine (USG <1.006)
      ii. hypotension leading to cardiovascular collapse
      iii. tachycardia
      iv. polydipsia (extreme thirst)
      v. hypernatremia
      vi. neurological changes
   b. Therapeutic Management
      i. water replacement
         1. D5W if IV replacement required
      ii. hormone replacement
         1. DDVAP (Desmopressin)
         2. Vasopressin
      iii. monitor urine output hourly and urine specific gravity
         1. report UO >200mL/hour
      iv. daily weight monitoring

Hyperthyroidism (Throtoxicosis)
1. Overview
   a. Excess secretion of thyroid hormone (TH) from thyroid gland resulting in **increased metabolic rate**
   b. Causes
      i. **Graves disease** (autoimmune reaction)
      ii. excess secretion of TSH, tumor, medication reaction
   c. Thyroid Storm (Thyroid Crisis)
      i. extreme hyperthyroidism (life threatening) due to infection, stress, trauma
         1. febrile state, tachycardia, HTN, tremors, seizures
2. NCLEX® Points
   a. Assessment

i. ↑T3, T4, free T4, ↓TSH, positive radioactive uptake scan
ii. goiter
iii. bulging eyes
iv. Cardiac
    1. tachycardia, HTN, palpitations
v. Neurological
    1. hyperactive reflexes, emotional instability, agitation, hand tremor
vi. Sensory
    1. **exophthalmos** (Graves disease), blurred vision, heat intolerance
vii. Integumentary
    1. fine thin hair
viii. Reproductive
    1. amenorrhea, decreased libido
ix. Metabolic
    1. increased metabolic rate, weight loss

3. Therapeutic Management
   a. provide rest in a cool quiet environment
   b. antithyroid medications (PTU, propylthiouracil)
   c. cardiac monitoring
   d. maintain patent airway
   e. provide eye protection
      i. regular eye exams
      ii. moisturize eyes
   f. Radioactive Iodine 131
      i. taken up by thyroid gland and destroys some thyroid cells over 6-8 weeks
         1. avoid with pregnancy
         2. monitor lab values for hypothyroidism
   g. Surgical removal
      i. monitor airway
         1. assess for obstruction, stridor, dysphagia
         2. have tracheotomy equipment available
      ii. maintain in semi-Fowlers position
      iii. assess surgical site for bleeding
      iv. monitor for hypocalcemia
         1. have calcium gluconate available
      v. minimal talking during immediate post operative period

Hypothyroidism
   1. Overview
      a. hyposecretion of TH resulting in decreased metabolic rate
      b. Myxedema coma
         i. lifethreatening state of decreased thyroid production
         ii. coma result of acute illness, rapid cessation of medication, hypothermia
   2. NCLEX® Points
      a. Assessment
         i. think HYPOmetabolic state

   ii. Cardiovascular
      1. bradycardia, anemia, hypotension
  iii. Gastrointestinal
      1. constipation
  iv. Neurological
      1. lethargy, fatigue, weakness, muscle aches, parethesias
   v. Integumentary
      1. goiter, dry skin, loss of body hair
  vi. Metabolic
      1. cold intolerance, anorexia, weight gain, edema, **hypoglycemia**

3. Therapeutic Management
   a. cardiac monitoring
   b. maintain open airway
   c. monitor medication therapy (overdose with thyroid medications possible)
   d. medication therapy
      i. levothyroxine (Synthroid)
   e. assess thyroid hormone levels
   f. IV fluids
   g. monitor and administer glucose as needed

Addison's Disease vs Cushing's Disease

Body System	Addison's (Hypo)	Cushing's (Hyper)
Cardiovascular	Hypotension, tachycardia	Hypertension, signs of CHF
Metabolic	Weight loss	Moon face, buffalo hump
Integumentary	Hyperpigmentation (bronze)	Fragile, striae abdomen and thighs
Electrolytes	Hyperkalemia, hypercalcemia, hyponatremia, hypoglycemia	Hypokalemia, hypocalcemia, hypernatremia, hyperglycemia

Addison's Disease
1. Overview
   a. **hyposecretion** of adrenal cortex hormones
   b. decreased levels of glucocorticoids and mineralcorticoids leads to hyponatremia, hyperkalemia, hypoglycemia, decreased vascular volume, fatal if untreated
2. NCLEX® Points
   a. Assessment
      i. review chart above

        ii. think HYPO secretion of adrenal hormones (steroids)
- b. Therapeutic Management
  - i. monitor vital signs
  - ii. monitor electrolytes (potassium, sodium, calcium)
  - iii. monitor glucose
    1. treat low blood sugar
  - iv. administer replacement adrenal hormones as needed
  - v. lifelong medication therapy needed
- c. Addisonian Crisis
  - i. caused by acute exacerbation of Addison's Disease
  - ii. causes severe electrolyte disturbances
  - iii. monitor electrolytes and cardiovascular status closely
  - iv. administer adrenal hormones as ordered

Cushing's Disease

1. Overview
   a. **hypersecretion** of glucocorticoids leading to **elevated cortisol levels**
   b. greater incidence in women
   c. life threatening if untreated
2. NCLEX® Points
   a. see chart above
   b. ↑cortisol, Na+, glucose, ↓K+ and Ca++
3. Therapeutic Management
   a. monitor electrolytes and cardiovascular status
   b. provide skin care and meticulous wound care
   c. provide for client safety
   d. adrenalectomy (surgical removal of adrenal gland)
   e. protect client from infection
   f. often caused by tumor on adrenal gland or pituitary gland

Diabetes Mellitus

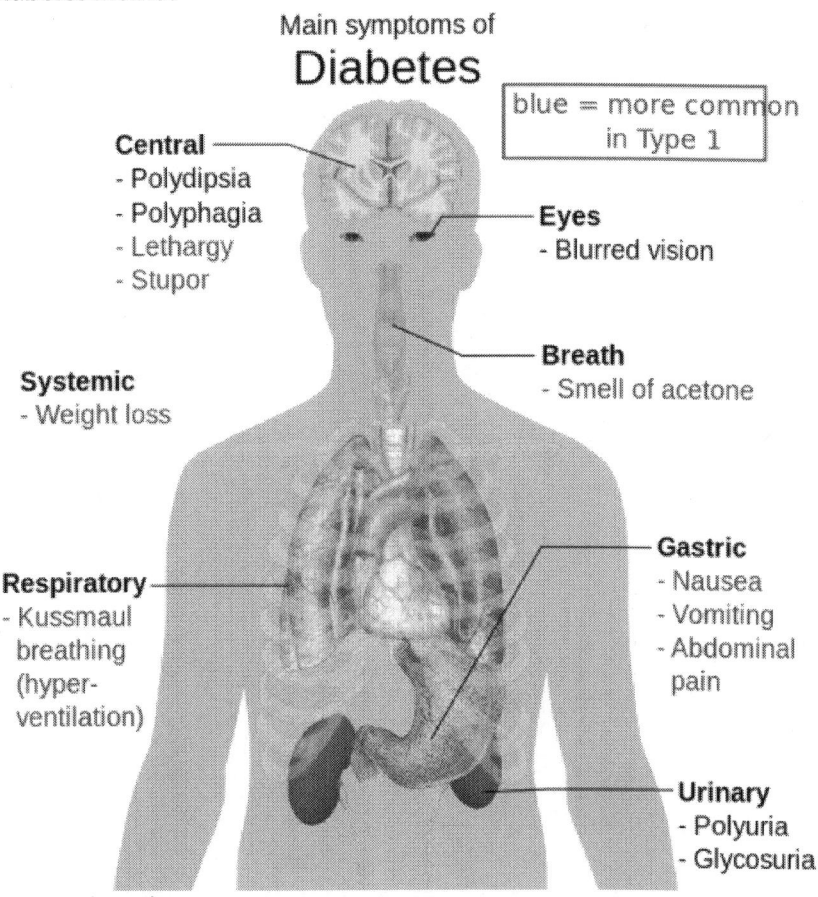

Main symptoms of
Diabetes

blue = more common in Type 1

Central
- Polydipsia
- Polyphagia
- Lethargy
- Stupor

Eyes
- Blurred vision

Breath
- Smell of acetone

Systemic
- Weight loss

Respiratory
- Kussmaul breathing (hyper-ventilation)

Gastric
- Nausea
- Vomiting
- Abdominal pain

Urinary
- Polyuria
- Glycosuria

1. Overview
   a. pancreatic disorder resulting in insufficient or lack of insulin production leading to elevated blood sugar
      i. **Type I (insulin dependent/juvenile-onset):** immune disorder, body attacks insulin producing beta cells with resulting **Ketosis** (result of ketones in blood due to gluconeogenesis from fat)
      ii. **Type II (insulin resistant/adult-onset):** beta cells do not produce enough insulin or body becomes resistant

2. NCLEX® Points
   a. Assessment
      i. 3 P's
         1. polyuria, polydipsia, polyphagia
      ii. elevate BS
      iii. blurred vision
      iv. elevated HgbA1C
      v. non healing wounds
      vi. neuropathy
      vii. inadequate circulation
      viii. End organ damage is a major concern due to damage to vessels
         1. coronary artery disease
            a. HTN, cerebrovascular disease
         2. retinopathy
   b. Therapeutic Management
      i. Insulin
         1. required for type I and for type II when diet and exercise do not control BS
         2. assess for and teach the patient regarding peak action time for various insulins
            a. only administer short acting insulins IV
         3. study onset times and peak times for insulins
         4. do not use expired insulin
         5. do not use a vial that appears cloudy (NPH exception)
         6. Mixing regular and NPH
            a. clear (regular) before cloudy (NPH)
            b. inject air needed into NPH, remove needle, inject air needed into regular, remove regular, remove NPH

  ii. patient should monitor BS before, during, and after exercise

  iii. patient should use protective footwear to prevent injury

  iv. infections and wounds should receive meticulous care

  v. foot care

   1. feet should be kept dry

   2. footwear should always be worn

   3. should not wear tight fitting socks

  vi. sick day

   1. continue to check blood sugars and **do not** withhold insulin

   2. monitor for ketones in urine

  vii. 15 rule

   1. if BS are low administer 15 gram CHO (5 lifesavers, 6 oz juice) recheck BS in 15 min

  viii. Complications

   1. lipoatrophy

    a. loss of subq fat at injection site (alternate injection sites)

   2. lipohypertrophy

    a. fatty mass at injection site

   3. Dawn phenomenon

    a. reduced insulin sensitivity between 5-8am

    b. evening administration may help

   4. Somogyi phenomenon

    a. night time hypoglycemia results in rebound hyperglycemia in the morning hours

Hyperglycemic Hyperosmolar Nonketotic Syndrome (HHNS)
1. Overview
    a. severe hyperglycemia without ketosis or acidosis
    b. most often with type II
    c. HHNS does not require the breakdown of fats for energy preventing ketosis. With HHNS enough insulin is available to breakdown carbs for energy.
2. NCLEX® Points
    a. Assessment
        i. gradual onset
            1. infection, stress, dehydration
        ii. altered LOC, dry mucous membranes
        iii. BS >600 mg/dL
        iv. negative ketones
        v. ↑ BUN and creatinine
    b. Therapeutic Management
        i. determine cause
        ii. replace fluids - may resolve hyperglycemia
        iii. insulin therapy
        iv. monitor neurological status
        v. treat electrolyte imbalances

Diabetic Ketoacidosis (DKA)
1. Overview
    a. severe insulin deficiency associated with type I diabetes
    b. leads to the breakdown of fats into glucose resulting in ketones
2. NCLEX® Points
    a. Assessment
        i. sudden onset
            1. infection, stress
        ii. fruity breath
        iii. ketones in urine
        iv. hyperglycemia
        v. dehydration
        vi. acidosis (pH <7.35)

     1. fats are broken down into glucose, ketones are by product of fat breakdown , ketones are acidic, potassium leaves the cell in attempt to compensate for acidemia

     2. http://www.eric.vcu.edu/home/resources/consults/Hyperkalemia.pdf

   vii. Kussmaul's respirations

   viii. hyperkalemia

   ix. ↑BUN and creatinine

   x. monitor for altered LOC - cerebral edema can occur with fluid shift

  b. Therapeutic Management

   i. treat dehydration - with hyperglycemia water moves out of cells

   ii. intensive insulin therapy

   iii. monitor potassium

   iv. assess for and treat acidosis

     1. helpful to assess anion gap vs pH alone as pH takes into account respiratory effects view more here: http://www.merckmanuals.com/professional/endocrine-and-metabolic-disorders/diabetes-mellitus-and-disorders-of-carbohydrate-metabolism/diabetic-ketoacidosis-dka

NCLEX® Cram - Metabolic and Endocrine Disorders

 1. Endocrine system

  a. hypothalamus

  b. pituitary gland (anterior/posterior)

  c. pineal gland

  d. thyroid gland

  e. parathyroid gland

  f. adrenal glands

g. pancreas

h. gonads

2. Endocrine system cheat sheet

Hormone	Gland	Under Production Syndrome	Over Production Syndrome
GH	anterior pituitary		acromegaly
ADH	posterior pituitary	diabetes insipidus	SIADH
T3,T4	thyroid	myxedema coma	graves
PTH	parathyroid	hyperparathyroid	hypoparathyroid
Glucocorticoids: cortisol	adrenal	addisons	cushings
Insulin	pancreas	diabetes mellitus	

3. Pituitary Gland Hormones
   a. ACTH
   b. FSH
   c. GH
   d. LH
   e. Prolactin
   f. TSH
   g. Oxytocin
   h. ADH

4. Radioactive Iodine Test
   a. measures thyroid function by measuring how much iodine is absorbed
      i. ↑iodine = hyperthyroidism

5. Glucocorticoids
   a. Cortisol
   b. blunt effect of insulin, suppress inflammation and immune response

6. Thyroid scan should not be completed on pregnant clients

7. Glucose Tolerance Test
   a. high level of glucose ingested
   b. glucose checked 2 hours after

       c.   level >200 mg/dL suggests DM

8. HgbA1c
       a.   indicates average plasma glucose concentration over time
       b.   goal for diabetic clients is <7%

9. Transspehnoidal Hypophysectomy
       a.   removal of pituitary tumor
       b.   primary post operative concern is monitoring for nasal drainage
       c.   assess for CSF in drainage using Halo Test
            i.   blood in center with clear ring surrounding blood
       d.   client **should not use a straw**

10. Pheochromocytoma
       a.   tumor of the adrenal medulla
       b.   causes excessive secretion of adrenal medulla hormones (epinephrine and norepinephrine)
       c.   HTN, palpitations, hyperglycemia, weight loss
       d.   avoid stimulation and provide constant cardiac monitoring
       e.   may need adrenalectomy

11. Parathyroid Disorders
       a.   think calcium
       b.   Hypoparathyroid = hypocalcemia
            i.   Trousseau's and Chvostek's signs

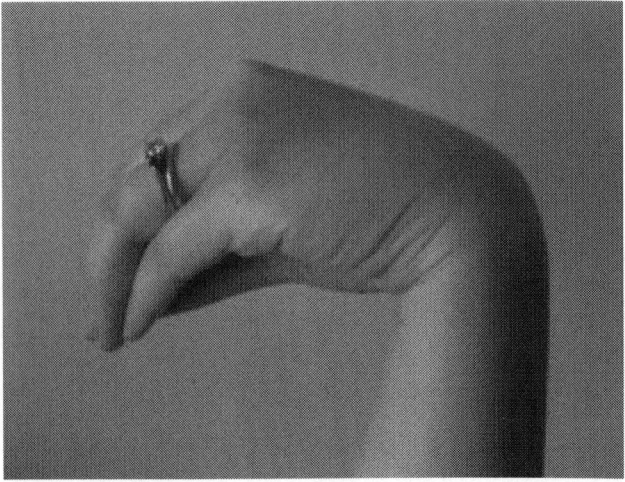

        ii.   provide calcium supplementation
       iii. provide vitamin D which aids in calcium absorption
  c. Hyperparathyroid = hypercalcemia
        i.   monitor for bone deformities
       ii. renal calculi

Osteoporosis

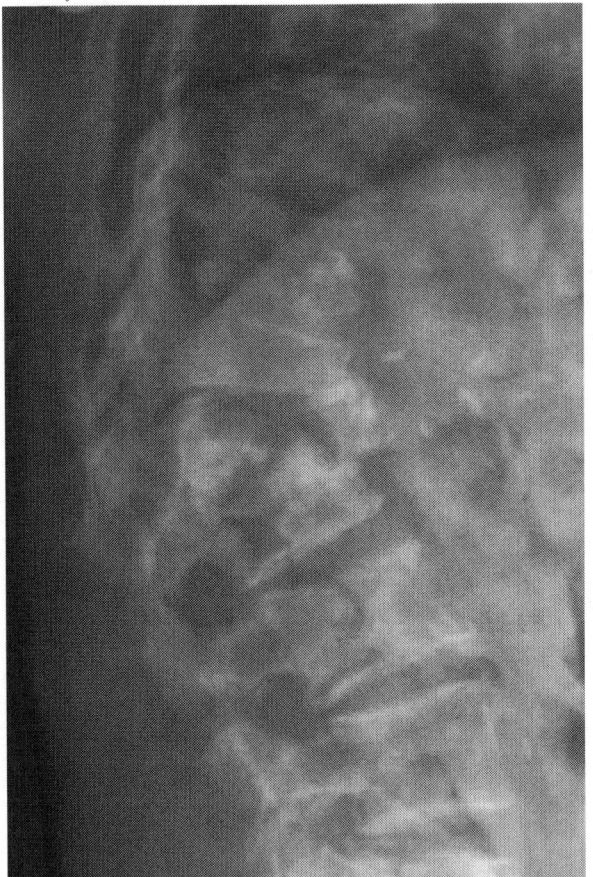

Clients with osteoporosis experience frequent fractures

1. Overview
   a. bone demineralization leading to ↓bone mass
   b. bone resorption occurs faster than formation leading to Ca loss and porous bones
   c. more common in women due to ↓ estrogen
   d. high risk for factures
2. NCLEX® Points
   a. Assessment
      i. steroid use
      ii. female

        iii. ↓Ca intake

        iv. Kyphosis of spine

        v. bone pain

        vi. fractures of pelvis or hip

  b. Therapeutic Management

        i. Ca+ intake and supplementation

        ii. Vitamin D intake

        iii. Weight bearing exercise

        iv. provide for a hazard free environment

        v. assistive devices

        vi. Medications

            1. alendronate (Fosamax)

            2. risendronate (Actonel)

            3. 30 minutes prior to eating

Osteoarthritis (Degenerative Joint Disease)

1. Overview

  a. progressive disorder of articulating joins

  b. affects weight-bearing joints and joints that receive a lot of stress (hands)

  c. Risk factors

        i. age, joint use, genetics

2. NCLEX® Points

  a. Assessment

        i. joint pain relieved with rest

        ii. Heberden's nodes and Bouchard's nodes

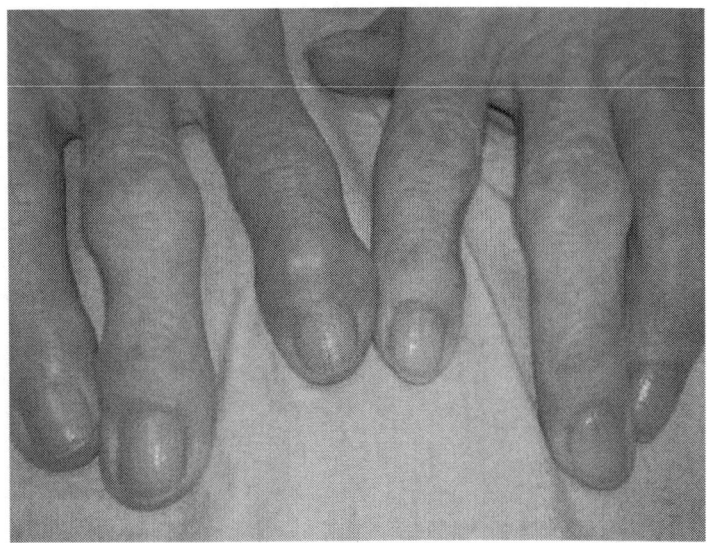

    iii. difficulty standing up after sitting

    iv. crepitus in joints (grating sensation)

  b. Therapeutic Management

    i. administer pain medications

     1. topical agents

     2. NSAIDs

     3. muscle relaxants

    ii. corticosteroid injections

    iii. heat/cold applications

    iv. schedule rest periods

Gout

 1. Overview

  a. urate crystals deposit in joints and body tissues

  b. Hyperuricemia caused by ↑ purine synthesis, dietary intake, heredity, ↓ renal excretion of uric acid, alcohol intake

 2. NCLEX® Points

  a. Assessment

    i. painful joint inflammation and swelling

  ii. **Tophi**: nodules in skin

  iii. pruritus

  iv. renal calculi

 b. Therapeutic Management

  i. Avoid purines

   1. organ meat

   2. wine

   3. aged cheese

  ii. adequate fluid intake

  iii. bed rest during exacerbations

  iv. Medications

   1. anti-inflammatories

   2. antihyperuricemic: allopurinal (Zyloprim)

Rheumatoid Arthritis

1. Overview
   a. **Chronic** and **systemic** inflammatory disorder leading to weakened joints, dislocation, and deformity
2. NCLEX® Points
   a. Assessment
      i. inflammation of joints
      ii. joint stiffness
      iii. spongy joints
      iv. ↑ESR
      v. + rheumatoid factor
      vi. joint deformities
      vii. anemia
3. Therapeutic Management
   a. range-of-motion activities
   b. scheduled rest times
   c. heat/cold therapy
   d. paraffin baths
   e. assess clients reaction to body changes
   f. joint replacement possible (arthroplasty)
   g. medications
      i. NSAIDs
      ii. DMARDs

     1. Disease Modifying Antirheumatic
      Drug
       a. slow progression of
        disease
    iii. glucocorticoids

NCLEX® Cram - Musculoskeletal Disorders
  1. Arthroscopy post procedure care
    a. assess neurovascular function
  2. Bone resorption increases with age
  3. Monitor site post biopsy for swelling, hematoma or pain
  4. Strain - excessive stretching of muscle
  5. Sprain - excessive stretching of ligament
    a. RICE
      i. Rest
      ii. Ice
      iii. Compression
      iv. Elevation

6. Types of fractures

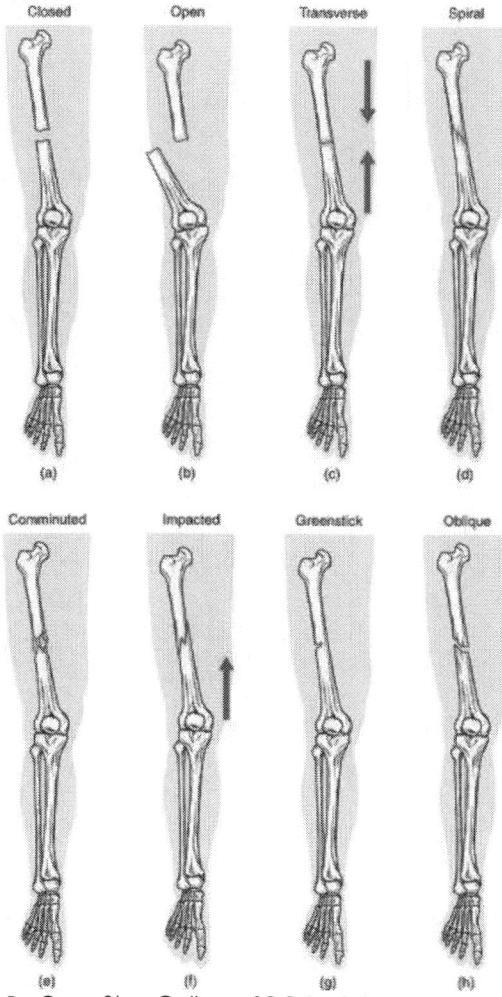

7. Traction
   a. force applied in opposite direction to immobilize fracture
   b. insure the body is properly aligned
   c. Buck's Traction

            i.   allow weights to hang from bed do not
                 set them on floor
        d. skeletal traction - uses pins inserted into bones
            i.   meticulous pin care required
        e. Weights should not be moved by anyone
8. Casts
        a. monitor extremity for swelling, pain, discoloration,
            loss of sensation, and pulse
9. Fat Embolism
        a. risk with long bone fractures
        b. originates in bone marrow and move into blood
            stream
        c. patient may become tachycadiac and
            hypotensive
        d. restless and tachypnea
        e. emergent intervention is required
10. Compartment Syndrome
        a. increased pressure within a body compartment
            usually with the arm or leg following trauma
            (fractures and crush injuries)
        b. results in insufficient blood supply to the muscles
            and nerves
        c. emergent surgery required to prevent loss of limb
        d. Assessment
            i.   tissue becomes pale
            ii.   loss of sensation distal to injury
            iii. pulseless
        e. Fasciaotomy required to relieve pressure
11. Crutches
        a. Going up Stairs
            i.   tripod position
            ii.   move unaffected leg up first
            iii. move crutches and affected leg up next
        b. Going down Stairs
            i.   move crutches down first
            ii.   move affected leg down next
12. Amputation
        a. Phantom Pain

       i. client has sensation of pain in amputated extremity
      ii. can be treated with analgesics
     iii. normal finding

13. Cane
    a. Stand on affected side of client
    b. hold cane on unaffected side
    c. canes and crutches should have rubber stoppers on the bottom
14. Hip Replacement
    a. proper body alignment must be observed postop
    b. monitor for fat embolism
    c. monitor wound and dressing for excessive drainage
15. Osteoporisis makes the client at risk for pathologic factures
16. Bone Scan
    a. client should drink adequate fluids to flush dye from system
17. Vitamin D aids in Calcium absorption
18. Insure a safe environment for clients using walkers, canes, and crutches

Immunological Disorders

Anaphylaxis
1. Overview
    a. Severe allergic reaction with rapid onset with massive histamine release from damaged cells
    b. Life threatening if untreated
2. NCLEX® Points
    a. Assessment
        i. hives
        ii. angioedema (facial swelling)
        iii. respiratory complications
        iv. cardiac arrest
        v. hypotension
        vi. skin flushing
    b. Therapeutic Management
        i. assess client for allergies
        ii. assess respiratory and cardiovascular status
        iii. administer epinephrine
        iv. administer oxygen
        v. administer antihistamines
        vi. provide fluids as needed

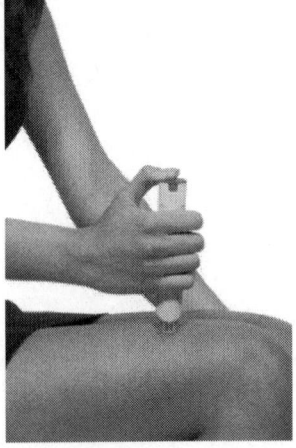

Systemic Lupus Erythematosus (SLE)

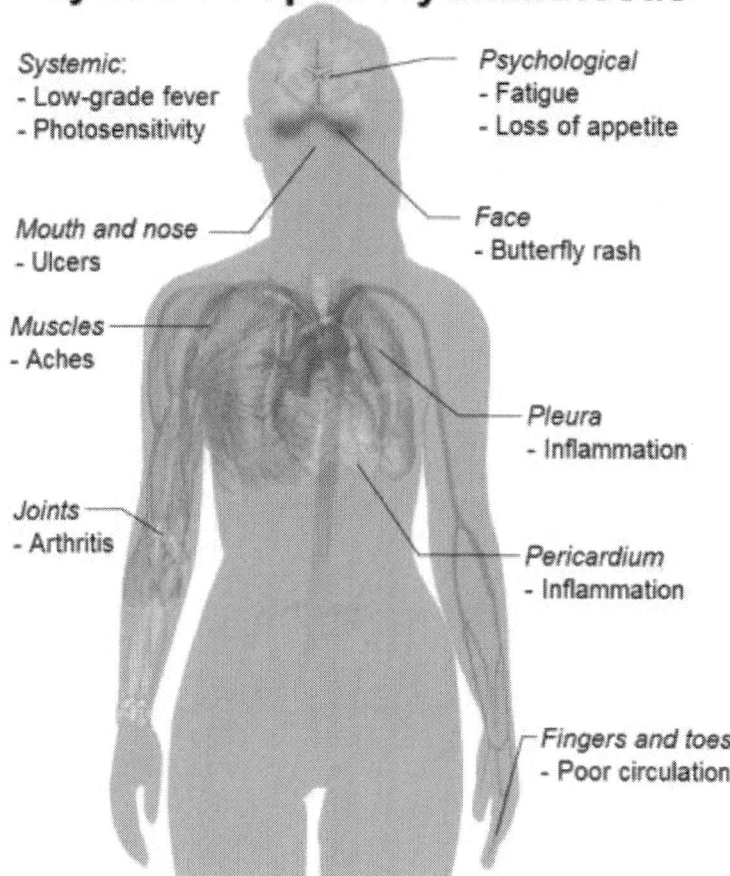

Most common symptoms of

Systemic lupus erythematosus

Systemic:
- Low-grade fever
- Photosensitivity

Psychological
- Fatigue
- Loss of appetite

Mouth and nose
- Ulcers

Face
- Butterfly rash

Muscles
- Aches

Pleura
- Inflammation

Joints
- Arthritis

Pericardium
- Inflammation

Fingers and toes
- Poor circulation

1. Overview
   a. progressive systemic inflammatory disease resulting in major organ system failure
   b. immune system "hyperactive" attacks healthy tissue
   c. no known cure
2. NCLEX® Points
   a. Assessment
      i. assess for precipitating factors

1. UV light
2. infection
3. stress
    ii. arthritis
    iii. weakness
    iv. photosensitivity
    v. Butterfly rash
    vi. ↑ESR and C Reactive Protein
b. Therapeutic Management
    i. assess respiratory status
    ii. assess end organ function
    iii. plan rest periods
    iv. identify triggers
    v. refer to dietitian for dietary assistance
    vi. Medications
        1. Glucocorticoids
        2. NSAIDs
        3. cyclophosamide (immunosupressive agent)

Acquired Immunodeficiency Syndrome (AIDS)

1. Overview
    a. Viral disease caused by HIV leading to spectrum of conditions
    b. Interferes with and destroys T4 cells making patient more susceptible to infections (TB, pneumonia, cancers, pneumonia)
2. NCLEX® Points
    a. Assessment
        i. Wasting syndrome
        ii. skin breakdown
        iii. frequent infections
        iv. stomatitis
        v. dehydration
        vi. malnutrition
        vii. leukopenia (↓WBCs)
        viii. Kaposi's sarcoma
            1. tumor caused by herpes virus

2. purple/red lesions on skin and organs
   b. Therapeutic Management
      i. respiratory support
      ii. nutritional support
         1. small frequent meals
         2. premedicate to avoid nausea
         3. provide favorite foods
      iii. monitor fluid and electrolyte balance
      iv. assess for infection
      v. provide skin care
      vi. initiate strict precautions and observe hand hygiene
      vii. conserve energy

Lyme Disease
1. Overview
   a. infection caused by tick bite
2. NCLEX® Points
   a. Assessment
      i. occur in three stages
      ii. flu-like symptoms
      iii. joint pain
      iv. neurological deficits
   b. Therapeutic Management
      i. remove tick
      ii. client should use bur spray prior to going outside
      iii. antibiotics must be taken as prescribed for the entire course
      iv. blood test can confirm diagnosis

NCLEX® Cram - Immunological Disorders
1. Innate Immunity
   a. present at birth
2. Acquired Immunity
   a. adaptive
      i. mother's antibodies
   b. active
      i. immunizations
3. Skin test
   a. discontinue taking antihistamines prior to test
4. assess all patient for latex allergy
5. clients with immunodeficiency are at a high risk for infection
6. patients who receive a transplant will have to take immunosuppressants for life
7. assess transplant patients closely for signs of rejection

Integumentary Disorders

Herpes Zoster (Shingles)
1. Overview
    a. viral infection seen in elderly individuals with a history of chicken pox
    b. occurs during immunocompromised state
    c. contagious to all individuals
2. NCLEX® Points
    a. vesicular rash
    b. fatigue, malaise, fever
3. Therapeutic Management
    a. isolation
    b. assess infection
    c. client may experience Bell's palsy
        i. assess neurological status
    d. Oatmeal bath may relieve itching
    e. Medications
        i. antivirals
        ii. NSAIDs
        iii. Shingles vaccination for elderly patients

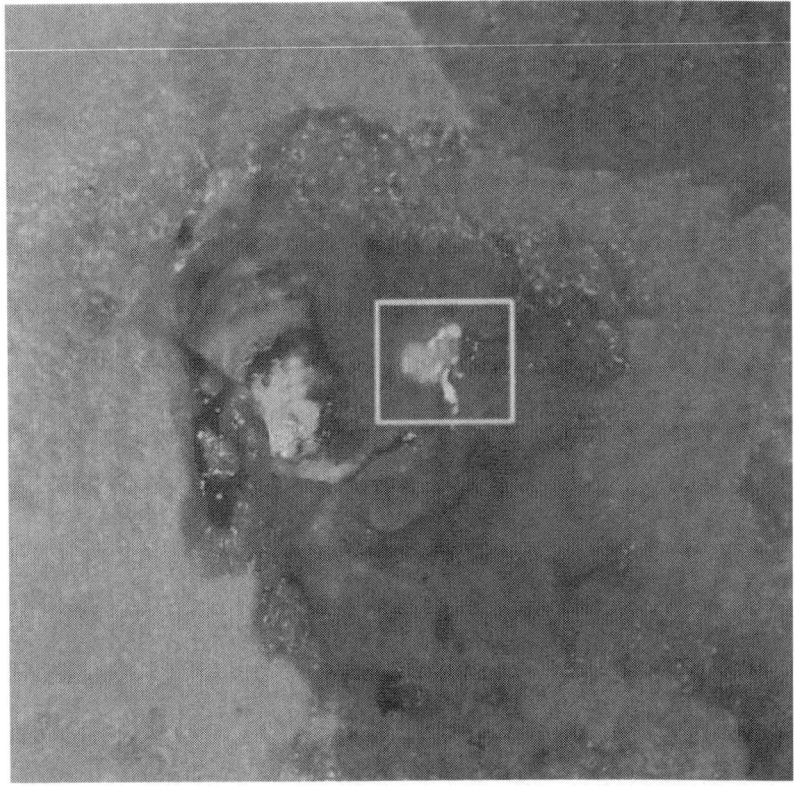

1. Overview
    a. excavations in the skin varying in size
    b. occur due to compression of tissue for extended period of time
2. NCLEX® Points
    a. Assessment
        i. Stage I
            1. skin is intact
            2. non blanchable redness
        ii. Stage II
            1. partial thickness loss of skin
        iii. Stage III
            1. full thickness skin loss extending to the dermis and subcutaneous tissue

          iv.   Stage IV
1. full thickness skin loss exposing bone and muscle
2. undermining and tunneling
3. eschar may be present

          v.   Deep Tissue Injury
1. subcutaneous tissue injury underneath skin

          vi. Unstageable
1. wound is covered by eschar or slough
2. unable to determine depth and thickness

b. Therapeutic Management
  i. **do not massage reddened area**
  ii. malnutrition, immobility, pressure are risk factors
  iii. assess patient skin integrity often
  iv. maintain skin dry
  v. turn patients q2h

Burns
1. NCLEX® Points
   a. Rule of 9s

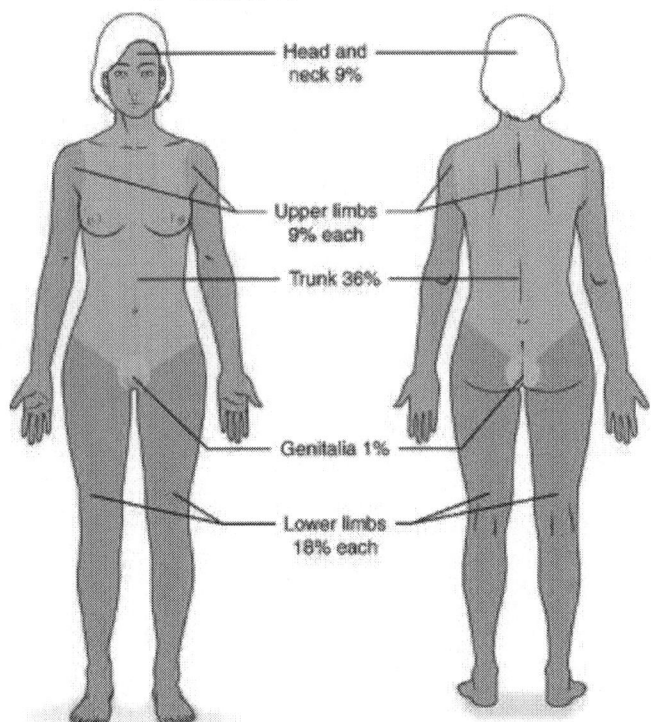

   b. Fluid resuscitation and infection prevention are the primary concern
   c. high calorie foods
   d. skin grafting
   e. monitor urine output - titrate fluid administration to urine output (30-50mL/hr)
   f. asses for edema

Skin Cancer
1. Overview
   a. abnormal cell growth
   b. excessive exposure to sun

2. NCLEX® Points
    a. Assessment
        i. Asymmetry
        ii. Border
        iii. Color
        iv. Diameter
        v. Elevation
    b. Therapeutic Management
        i. Biopsy to confirm diagnosis
        ii. instruct the client on risk factors
        iii. educate on how to monitor lesions

NCLEX® Cram - Integumentary Disorders

1. Petechiae
    a. small red spots that do not change color
2. keloid
    a. irregular darker area of scar often seen with African Americans
3. MRSA (Methicillin-Resistant Staphylococcus Aureus)
    a. contagious skin or wound infection that is spread by direct contact
    b. maintain standard and contact precautions
4. Frostbite
    a. rewarm with water and towels to salvage as much tissue as possible
5. Contact dermatitis
    a. skin inflammation due to allergic reaction
    b. Assessment
        i. vesicles, bullae, erythema, oozing, scaling
    c. Treatment
        i. topical corticosteroids
        ii. Burrow's solution
6. Stevens-Johnson Syndrome
    a. drug induced skin reaction leading to the epidermis separating from the dermis
    b. identify the cause, antibiotics, corticosteroids

Hematologic/Oncology Disorders

Anemia

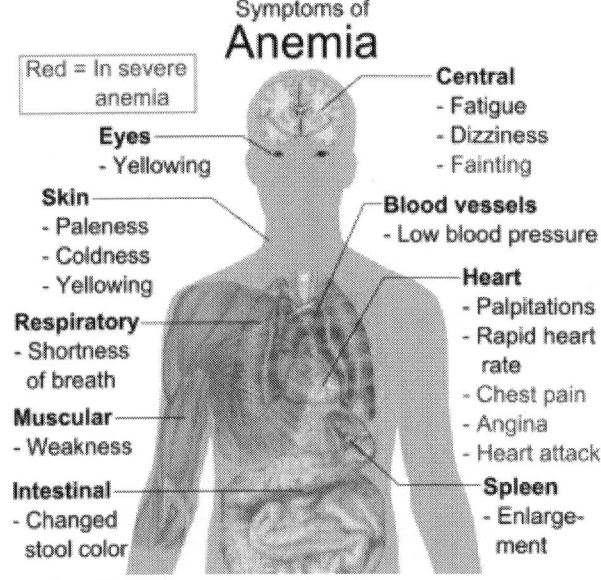

Symptoms of

Anemia

Red = In severe
anemia

Central
- Fatigue
- Dizziness
- Fainting

Eyes
- Yellowing

Skin
- Paleness
- Coldness
- Yellowing

Blood vessels
- Low blood pressure

Heart
- Palpitations
- Rapid heart
  rate
- Chest pain
- Angina
- Heart attack

Respiratory
- Shortness
  of breath

Muscular
- Weakness

Intestinal
- Changed
  stool color

Spleen
- Enlarge-
  ment

1. Overview
   a. ↓ in amount of RBCs or hemoglobin in blood, ↓ capacity of blood to carry oxygen
   b. Iron-Deficiency
      i. inadequate iron supply - 60% of anemias
   c. Pernicious
      i. Vitamin B12 deficiency
   d. Aplastic
      i. ↓ production of RBCs
2. NCLEX® Points
   a. Assessment
      i. pallor
      ii. weakness
      iii. cheilosis
      iv. spoonlike nails
      v. ↓MCV, MCH, Iron
      vi. Pica - craving clay and starch
      vii. Schillin test (for Pernicious anemia)
   b. Therapeutic Management
      i. assess for occult blood

ii.   monitory laboratory studies (Hgb, Hct)
iii. Increase iron intake in diet
     1.   green leafy vegetables
     2.   organ meat
iv. provide iron supplements
v.   administer Iron via Z-track method
vi. take iron on an empty stomach
vii. limit visitors to patients with aplastic anemia

Sickle Cell Disease

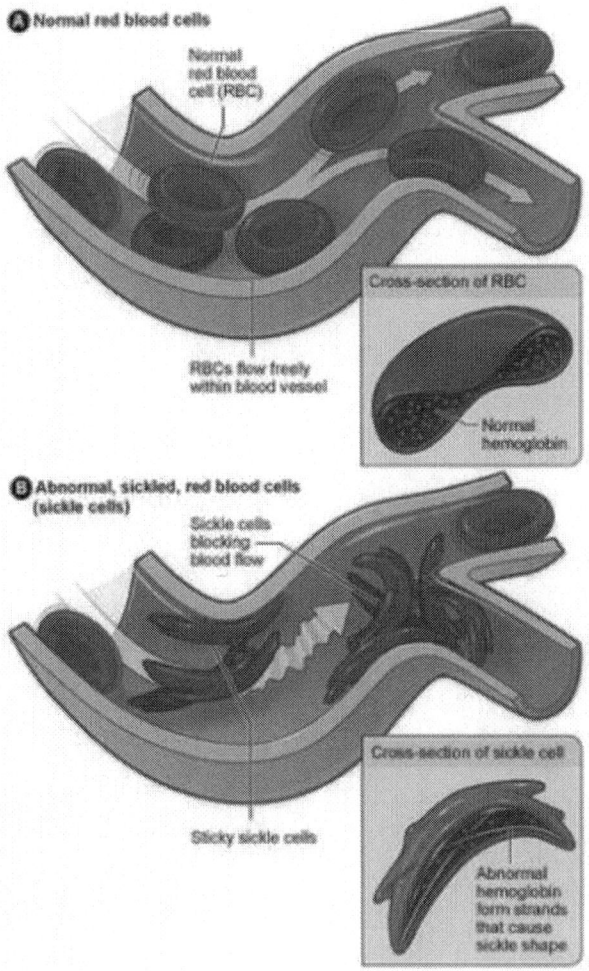

A Normal red blood cells

Normal red blood cell (RBC)

RBCs flow freely within blood vessel

Cross-section of RBC

Normal hemoglobin

B Abnormal, sickled, red blood cells (sickle cells)

Sickle cells blocking blood flow

Sticky sickle cells

Cross-section of sickle cell

Abnormal hemoglobin form strands that cause sickle shape

1. Overview
   a. hereditary disorder that affects the hemoglobin ability to carry oxygen leading to rigid, misshapen RBCs
   b. primarily affects African Americans by recessive trait
   c. can lead to sickle cell crisis due to hypoxia, exercise, high altitude, fever
2. NCLEX® Points

a. Assessment
    i. pallor
    ii. fatigue
    iii. severe pain

b. Therapeutic Management
    i. supplemental oxygen
    ii. increase fluid intake
    iii. provide analgesia
    iv. blood transfusion

Thrombocytopenia
1. Overview
    a. Decrease in circulating platelets (<100,000/mL)
    b. Causes
        i. decreased production
        ii. increased destruction
        iii. medication induced
2. NCLEX® Points
    a. Assessment
        i. ↓ platelet count
        ii. petechiae
        iii. bleeding (epistaxis, gi bleeding, melena, hematuria)
        iv. ↓Hgb, Hct
        v. monitor CBC
    b. Therapeutic Management
        i. platelet transfusions
        ii. Bleeding precautions
            1. avoid invasive procedures
            2. soft bristled toothbrush
            3. avoid medications that interfere with coagulation
            4. monitor for signs of bleeding
        iii. Diagnosis made via bone marrow aspiration

Disseminated Intravascular Coagulation (DIC)
1. Overview

      a. widespread activation of the clotting cascade that results in the formation of blood clots in the small blood vessels throughout the body, normal clotting is disrupted and severe bleeding and hemorrhage occurs

2. NCLEX® Points
   a. Assessment
      i. pallor
      ii. ecchymosis
      iii. hematomas
      iv. hemoptysis
      v. melena
      vi. occult blood in stool
      vii. dyspnea
      viii. chest pain
      ix. hematuria
      x. anxiety
      xi. confusion
      xii. prolonged aPTT, PT, and thrombin time
      xiii. ↓platelets
   b. Therapeutic Management
      i. determine and treat underlying cause immediately
      ii. replace clotting factors
      iii. initiate bleeding precautions
      iv. monitor I&O

Leukemia
1. Overview
   a. proliferation of abnormal, undeveloped WBCs
   b. diagnosed by blood tests and bone marrow biopsy
   c. characterized by type of WBC affected
      i. Acute lymphocytic leukemia (ALL)
         1. 2-4 years of age
      ii. Chronic lymphocytic leukemia (CLL)
         1. 50-70 years of age
      iii. Acute myelogenous leukemia (AML)
         1. peak at 60 years of age
      iv. Chronic myelogenous leukemia (CML)

1.   incidence increases with age

2. NCLEX® Points
   a. Assessment

Common symptoms of
Leukemia

Systemic
- Weight loss
- Fever
- Frequent infections

Lungs
- Easy shortness
  of breath

Muscular
- Weakness

Bones or joints
- Pain or
  tenderness

Psychological
- Fatigue
- Loss of appetite

Lymph nodes
- Swelling

Spleen and/or liver
- Enlargement

Skin
- Night sweats
- Easy bleeding
  and bruising
- Purplish
  patches
  or spots

   i. weight loss
   ii. fever
   iii. infections
   iv. pain in joints
   v. fatigue
   vi. night sweets
   vii. easy bleeding and bruising
   viii. ↑WBC CLL and CML
   ix. ↓WBC ALL and AML
   x. Philadelphia chromosome in majority of
      CML clients
   b. Therapeutic Management
       i. chemotherapy and radiation
       ii. apply pressure to biopsy site
       iii. initiate neutropenic precautions
       iv. initiate bleeding precautions

           v.   reverse isolation
                1.   gown
                2.   glove
                3.   sterilize all equipment
                4.   strict hand washing
                5.   no fresh fruits or flowers
          vi. avoid fatigue
                1.   plan activities to provide time for rest
         vii. instruct client on oral hygiene
                1.   rinse mouth with saline
                     a.   avoid lemon, alcohol base mouth wash

Lymphoma

1. Overview
   a. cancer or the lymphatic system
   b. classified by cell type many forms but Hodgkin's vs non-Hodgkin's (90% are non-Hodgkin's)
2. NCLEX® Points
   a. Assessment
      i. Reed-Sternberg cells - Hodgkins only
      ii. Positive biopsy
      iii. night sweets
      iv. fatigue
      v. enlarged liver, spleen, and lymph nodes
   b. Therapeutic Management
      i. Chemotherapy and/or radiation
      ii. assess for bleeding

NCLEX® Cram - Hematologic/Oncology Disorders

1. Warning signs of cancer
   a. CAUTION
      i. Change in bowel pattern
      ii. Unusual bleeding
      iii. Thickening of breast, testicle, skin
      iv. Indigestion
      v. Obvious change in mole
      vi. Nagging cough
2. Cancer Staging

      a. Stage 0: carcinoma in situ
      b. Stage I: local tumor growth
      c. Stage II: limited spreading
      d. Stage III: regional spreading
      e. Stage IV: metastasis
3. Testicular Cancer
      a. instruct client to perform monthly self examination
         i. best preformed after warm shower
4. Cervical Cancer
      a. women should have regular gynecological examinations with Pap smear testing

5. Breast Cancer
    a. metastisis can easily occur via the lymph nodes
    b. diagnosis is made via biopsy or tumor removal
    c. Risk Factors
        i. early menarche or late menopause
    d. BSE (Breast Self Examination)
        i. perform monthly 7-10 days after menses
    e. Do not perform blood pressure checks or invasive procedures on an arm that has had a mastectomy
6. Prostate Cancer
    a. men after 50 should have regular prostate examinations
    b. removal of the prostate gland can be achieved via Transurethral Resection of the Prostate (TURP)
7. Hemophilia A and B are X linked recessive traits carried by females and demonstrated in males
    a. leads to prolonged clotting times
8. Neutropenia
    a. WBC <2000/mm3
        i. observe reverse isolation
        ii. observe strict hand hygiene
        iii. no fresh fruits, vegetables, or flowers

Eye, Ear, Nose and Throat Disorders

Strabismus
1. Overview
   a. eyes do not properly align with each other
   b. due to lack of ocular muscle coordination
2. NCLEX® Points
   a. Assessment
      i. cover-uncover test
      ii. squinting
   b. Therapeutic Management
      i. patch good eye 1-2 hours daily
      ii. surgical repair

Amblyopia
1. Overview
   a. also referred to as lazy eye involves decreased vision in an otherwise normal appearing eye
2. NCLEX® Points
   a. signs of visual impairment
   b. diagnosed by optometrist
3. Therapeutic Management
   a. corrective lenses
   b. cover good eye a few hours daily

Glaucoma

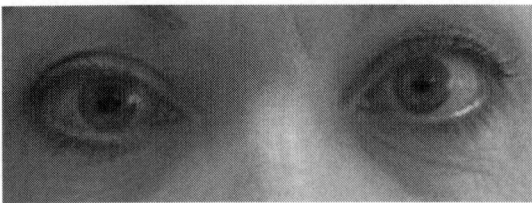

By James Heilman, MD (Own work) [CC BY-SA 3.0 (http://creativecommons.org/licenses/by-sa/3.0) or GFDL (http://www.gnu.org/copyleft/fdl.html)], via Wikimedia Commons
1. Overview
   a. Optic nerve damage caused by increased intra ocular pressure
   b. Two main categories
      i. Open-angle
         1. painless

                2. develops slowly
                3. no symptoms until advanced

        ii. Closed-angle (medical emergency)
                1. sudden eye pain
                2. redness
                3. vomiting
                4. sudden spike in intraocular
                   pressure
    2. NCLEX® Points
        a. Medication
                i. miotic drugs to constrict pupils
        b. requires lifelong drug therapy
        c. avoid medication that dilate pupils
                i. atropine
                ii. mydriatics
        d. institute safety measures for poor vision especially
           at night and in low light

Cataracts
    1. Overview
        a. Clouding of the lens leading to decrease in vision
        b. risks include age, smoking, injury, DM
    2. NCLEX® Points
        a. Assessment
                i. vision changes
                ii. loss of color vision
                iii. clouding of pupil
                iv. halos
                v. absence of red reflex
        b. Therapeutic Management
                i. surgery for removal of lens one eye at a
                   time
                ii. patient safety is a priority
                iii. assist with ADLs
                iv. instruct client on eye protection

Detached Retina
    1. Overview
        a. retina peels away from underlying support tissue

b. medical emergency
2. NCLEX® Points
   a. Assessment
      i. sensation of curtain covering vision field
      ii. painless
      iii. gray retina
   b. Therapeutic Management
      i. the goal is to find and repair retinal breaks
      ii. lay client with affected side dependent
      iii. protect client from injury

Ménière's Disease
1. Overview
   a. disorder of the inner ear affecting hearing and balance
2. NCLEX® Points
   a. Assessment
      i. vertigo
      ii. tinnitus
      iii. hearing loss
      iv. head ache
   b. Therapeutic Management
      i. ↓Na intake
         1. ↑Na intake can exacerbate symptoms
      ii. bedrest
      iii. cochlear implant
      iv. endolymphatic sac decompression: create shunt for fluid drainage

NCLEX® Cram - Eye, Ear, Nose and Throat Disorders
1. Myopia
   a. nearsightedness
2. Hyporopia
   a. farsightedness
3. Closed Angle Glaucoma
   a. sudden eye pain with N/V
4. Never remove a penetrating object from the eye
5. Chemical splash

       a.   flush the eyes for 15-20 minutes
6.   Never use ear candles to remove cerumen
7.   Rinne Test
       a.   hearing test used to evaluate unilateral hearing loss
       b.   vibrating tuning fork on mastoid bone
8.   Weber Test
       a.   used to detect unilateral conductive hearing loss
       b.   vibrating tuning fork placed in middle of forehead

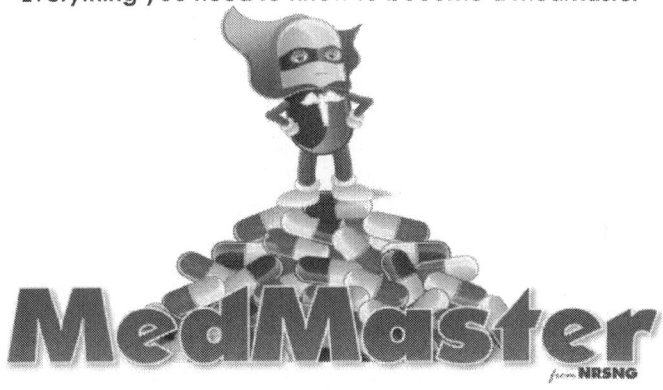

Nursing Case Studies
15 Med-Surg Case Studies for Nursing Students
NRSNG.com | NursingStudentBooks.com
Jon Haws RN CCRN
Sandra Haws RD CNSC
©TazKai LLC 2015

Nursing
Case Studies

Pneumothorax
Pancreatitis
Acidosis
CABG
STEMI
Sepsis
DKA
Stroke
Seizures
COPD
ESRD
CHF
More . . .

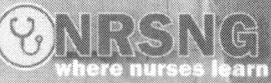

NRSNG
where nurses learn

Introduction

Nursing is a complex field. It is both an art and a science.

The way in which we talk with and care for our patients requires art.

Understanding and treating complex physiologic conditions is a science.

Knowing how to best care for complex patients requires intense studying and focus. This book provides 15 case studies on some of the most common and most complex maladies that our patients face.

Learning how to address these issues will help you in your studies, on the NCLEX®, and in your practice as a nurse.

The selection process for the 15 diseases covered in this book included drawing on my experience as a CCRN in a large metropolitan ICU, speaking with other nurses in various specialties, referring to a mountain of NCLEX® prep books, reviewing CCRN study materials, speaking with physicians, and reviewing NIH (National Institute of Health) data regarding the most commonly presenting conditions in hospitals.

My goal is that you become a highly knowledgeable, skilled, and caring practitioner.

This is not a ONE and DONE book. Spend time on the rationales. Use this book as a clinical reference and as a study guide for exams. Much effort and time was put into creating a book that will aid you in becoming the best nurse possible.

As you read the case studies reflect on the knowledge that you already have about the disease, as you read the questions refer to your notes and study materials to attempt to answer without reading the rationales. You can do this . . . nursing is hard . . . but it is the most rewarding career in the world.

Happy Nursing!

-Jon Haws RN CCRN

Diabetic Ketoacidosis

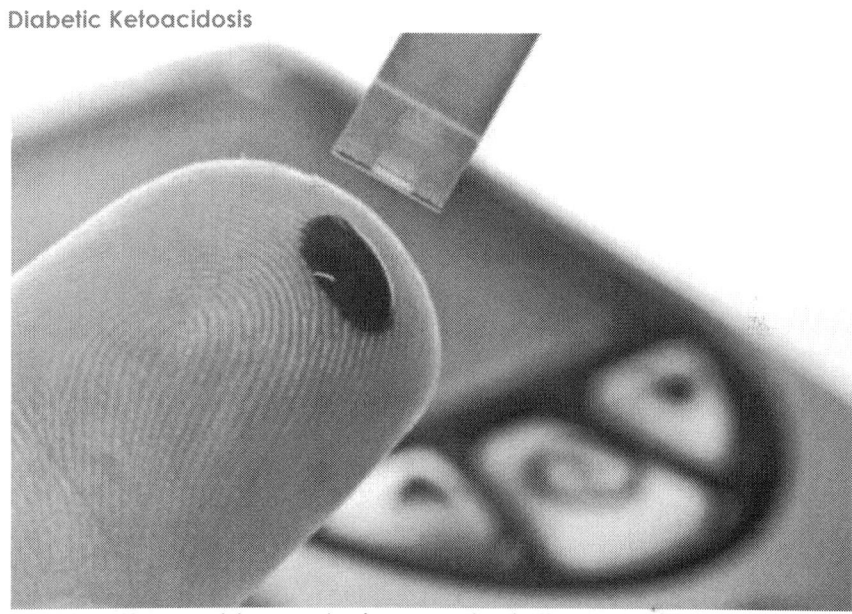

Mr. L. is a 58-year-old man who is recovering in the orthopedic unit of the hospital from a right total knee replacement of two days ago. Mr. L. has type I diabetes and was diagnosed with the condition at 12 years old. He has been managing his illness with blood glucose checks 4 times a day: before meals and once at bedtime. He currently takes Humulin-R on a sliding scale based on his glucose results. He weighs 315 lbs. and has developed osteoarthritis in both knees, requiring surgical replacement of the knee joint on the right side.

The nurse caring for Mr. L. enters his room at 8:15 am for a morning assessment. She finds Mr. L. lying in his bed awake, but his mental status is altered and there is a fruity odor to his breath. His vital signs are: HR 100 bpm, RR 32/minute, BP 116/78 mmHg. The nurse notes that his last blood glucose level was 156 mg/dL the previous night before bed and he received 2 units of insulin at that time, but he has not received his morning glucose check or any insulin yet today. A rapid bedside glucose check reveals a blood glucose level of 468 mg/dL. The nurse contacts the physician and upon further examination, Mr. L. is diagnosed with diabetic ketoacidosis.

1. Describe how diabetic ketoacidosis could develop in a patient who has undergone surgery.

2. Mr. L has an elevated respiratory rate that is classified as Kussmaul respirations. Explain this type of respiratory pattern.

Mr. L complains of feeling very thirsty and that he can't see very well because his vision is suddenly blurry. The nurse notes that he has a large amount of clear urine in his catheter bag. She takes a sample of urine and it tests positive for ketone bodies.

3. How does the body release ketones into the urine when DKA occurs?

4. Explain why Mr. L would have increased urinary output, blurred vision, and increased thirst.

The physician has given orders to administer 0.9% Sodium Chloride IV at 500 mL/hour for 1 hour, then 200 mL/hour for the next 4 hours. The nurse is to start a drip of Regular insulin at 0.1 mg/kg/hour. The physician has also added orders for laboratory work, including a metabolic profile and arterial blood gases. The metabolic panel results are: Na 135 mEq/L, K 3.2 mEq/L, Cl 95 mmol/L, Ca 8.5 mg/dL. The arterial blood gas results are as follows: pH 7.31, pCO2 20 mmHg, pO2 95 mmHg, HCO3 12 mmol/L.

5. What is the rationale for the IV fluids to be given at this rate?

6. Explain why the patient's potassium result is at the current level.

7. Based on the metabolic profile results, what is the next step that the nurse would most likely need to perform?

8. Explain why DKA would most likely produce these types of blood gas results.

An hour after the insulin was started, the nurse checks Mr. L's blood glucose levels and notes it has decreased to 208 mg/dL. He appears more comfortable and his vital signs are: HR 92 bpm, RR 22/minute, BP 116/70 mmHg, O2 saturation 95% on 2L of oxygen.

9. What should the nurse do next?

Rationale

Diabetic ketoacidosis is a condition that causes significant hyperglycemia and puts the body into a state of acidosis because of the production of ketones. It is more common in patients with type 1 diabetes when compared to those with type 2. DKA may be more likely to occur during times of infection or when increased levels of cortisol are secreted as a result of stress. Thus, the patient who has had surgery may be experiencing extra stress in the body or he could be developing an infection, which would cause the ketoacidosis. An essential goal of treatment is to manage the underlying cause of DKA to prevent it from recurring.

The patient with DKA is likely to have changes in mental status and complain of being thirsty; he may be diaphoretic and have increased urinary output as well as an increased respiratory rate and a fruity odor to the breath. Kussmaul respirations are a pattern of deep and rapid breathing as the body tries to get rid of excess carbon dioxide that has built up. During DKA, the body breaks down fat to use as energy instead of using glucose from the bloodstream. Ketones accumulate in the blood and the urine as a result of this fat breakdown, and the nurse may note elevated ketone bodies in laboratory results or with a urine dipstick test.

The severe hyperglycemia in this condition causes excess glucose and fluid to enter the urine, which significantly increases urinary output, causing polyuria and putting the patient at risk of dehydration. Mr. L is most likely suffering from fluid volume deficit and needs rapid IV replacement of fluid into the intravascular space to prevent complications, as well as intravenous insulin to counter the very high blood glucose levels. With insulin administration, potassium will move from the bloodstream and into the cells, which decreases the level of serum potassium as shown on exam. Because the patient is at risk of severe hypokalemia due to DKA, the nurse should administer IV potassium as replacement therapy if potassium levels are low and monitor for signs and symptoms of hypokalemia, including cardiac arrhythmias.

Mr. L is demonstrating metabolic acidosis, which can occur because of the increase in ketone bodies, which are acids that are created when the body tries to use energy from fat. The nurse should continue to monitor the patient's respiratory rate and provide supplemental oxygen to keep oxygen saturations within normal limits. With continued administration of intravenous insulin as treatment of DKA, the patient's blood glucose levels may quickly drop into the normal range. When this occurs, the nurse should administer glucose with the IV fluid to prevent Mr. L.'s blood glucose levels from dropping too rapidly and to minimize the potential for cerebral edema because of the significant change in serum glucose levels. The nurse will most likely need to continuously monitor the patient's fluid intake and should recheck the blood glucose levels frequently to ensure that they are within normal limits.

Congestive Heart Failure

Mrs. S., a 63-year-old patient who suffered a myocardial infarction last year, is in the cardiac rehabilitation center for follow-up after suffering from fatigue and shortness of breath; she complains of a "fluttering" feeling with her heartbeat and she has an occasional productive cough. Mrs. S. normally does not struggle with nighttime urination, but for the past month, she has had to get up to use the bathroom 2 to 3 times each night. She has gained 5 pounds in the past week.

1. Mrs. S.'s physician believes that she has developed congestive heart failure after having an MI last year. Which test would most likely be used to confirm the presence of CHF?

2. The nurse performs a physical assessment on Mrs. S. and checks her respiratory rate while listening to her lung sounds. If Mrs. S. has CHF, what signs would the nurse most likely notice when performing a respiratory assessment?

After diagnostic testing, Mrs. S. is diagnosed with congestive heart failure. Her physician prescribes oral Lasix for her to take every day to help with some of her symptoms and assists her with starting a program through cardiac rehabilitation where she can exercise on a routine basis and continue to be monitored by health professionals.

3. What types of tests would this patient undergo that would diagnose heart failure?

4. How does Lasix help with congestive heart failure symptoms?

5. What information should the nurse include with teaching Mrs. S. about taking a diuretic medication, such as Lasix?

6. In addition to regular exercise, what other types of lifestyle changes should Mrs. S. implement to control her symptoms of heart failure?

Mrs. S. has started taking Lasix and continues with cardiac rehabilitation. She has lost the recent weight she gained and is able to walk a little further than before when using the treadmill. She also does not get up as often during the night to use the bathroom when she takes her Lasix first thing in the morning. However, Mrs. S. still complains of a fluttering feeling in her chest and her blood pressure readings have been elevated. Her last BP at her appointment was 140/88 mmHg. The physician orders Captopril 50 mg po tid and has her come back to the clinic in 2 more weeks.

7. What type of drug is Captopril?

8. Why would this type of medication be prescribed for a patient with heart failure?

9. What information is most important for the nurse to give this patient when using this medication?

10. How would Mrs. S know if her medications are working to control her heart failure?

Rationale

Heart failure, sometimes referred to as congestive heart failure or CHF, is a condition in which the heart is unable to pump enough blood to keep up with the circulatory needs of the body. Heart failure develops because of various problems associated with cardiac function; some cases are caused by ventricular dysfunction, problems with the heart valves, or decreased cardiac contractility. When the heart cannot function properly because of heart failure, the person experiences decreased organ perfusion and may develop organ dysfunction and peripheral fluid accumulation.

Upon assessment, the patient with heart failure often has decreased activity tolerance and difficulties breathing. The nurse may note rales or crackles on auscultation of lung sounds because of increased fluid. Other signs or symptoms include peripheral edema, jugular venous distention, high blood pressure and cardiac arrhythmias or disorders of heart sounds as noted on auscultation. Heart failure is diagnosed by taking the patient's medical history and assessing signs and symptoms, as well as some diagnostic tests, such as ECG to assess cardiac rhythms, echocardiogram to look for changes in the heart's structure, and chest x-ray to look for extra fluid in the lungs.

Management of heart failure is done by getting rid of excess fluid in circulation, typically by administering a diuretic medication. A diuretic such as Lasix is used to get the body to excrete more fluid into the urine, where it can then be eliminated from the body through urination. Removal of excess fluid can then help the patient's activity tolerance and can reduce other symptoms of excess fluid volume, such as edema and wet lung sounds. When taking a diuretic such as Lasix, the nurse should be sure to instruct the client to take the drug in the morning; Lasix causes increased urinary output, which can be managed better during the day when the patient is awake. Taking Lasix in the evening may cause the patient to have to get up to use the bathroom more during the night. The nurse should also instruct the client about other lifestyle changes she can make to manage her heart failure, including decreasing sodium intake in the diet, weighing daily, restricting fluid intake to less than 2 L per day, participating in moderate amounts of exercise, and quitting smoking, if needed.

Although a diuretic medication can help with excess fluid associated with heart failure, the patient may also need to take other medications to improve heart function and to support the work of the heart, thus decreasing some of the effects of heart failure. Angiotensin-converting enzyme (ACE) inhibitor medications act as vasodilators to reduce blood pressure and to reduce the workload of the heart. Captopril, the drug prescribed for the patient in this example, is a type of ACE inhibitor. When giving the patient this drug, the nurse should ensure that the patient knows the effects of the drug and what signs or symptoms to look for to indicate that it is working. Captopril decreases blood pressure, so the patient should be taught about what to do if she feels lightheaded or dizzy or experiences other signs of hypotension. The patient can know that this drug is working to treat her heart failure if she is able to perform more activities without becoming short of breath, and if she experiences decreased dyspnea overall.

Ischemic stroke

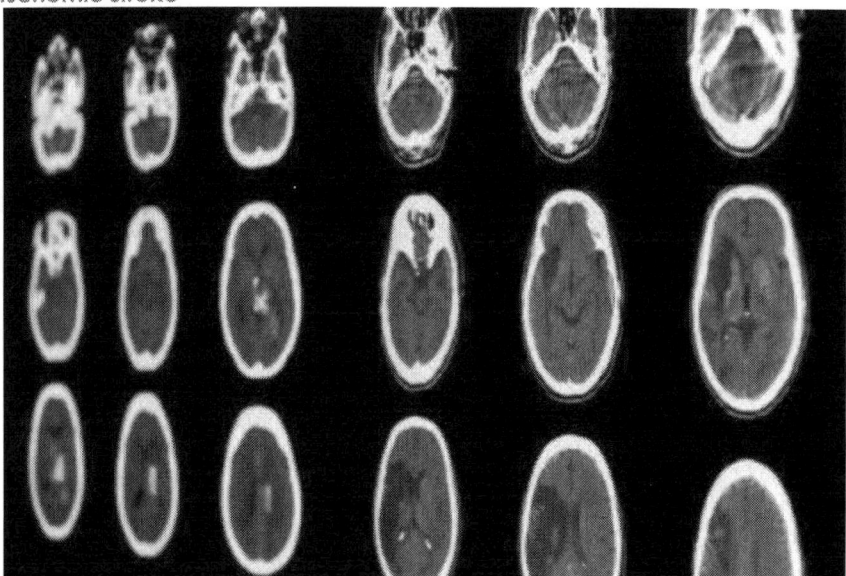

Mr. K is a 71-year-old male who has been brought in to the emergency department by his daughter, who was visiting his house for lunch and noticed that he seemed confused. Mr. K does not have a history of confusion, however, he lives alone and his daughter is concerned that he does not take care of himself. He has a medical history of type 2 diabetes and high cholesterol and he is a smoker. During the visit with his daughter, he had trouble walking and complained of feeling nauseated and dizzy. He told his daughter that he has had the hiccups for the past day but he cannot remember when he started feeling dizzy or ill. His daughter immediately brought him to the emergency department.

Upon exam, Mr. K complains of pain in his left arm and his left leg and he has left-sided weakness. He is unable to maintain his balance and requires assistance with getting into the bed. A rapid neurological assessment also reveals left-sided facial weakness and nystagmus. The nurse checks his vital signs and takes the following:
HR 88bpm, RR 18/minute, BP 142/90 mmHg, T 95.8°F. Based on his initial exam and symptoms, the physician believes that Mr. K may have suffered a stroke.

1. Based on the nurse's knowledge of how an ischemic stroke develops, which of Mr. K's risk factors would have most likely contributed to his condition and why?

2. Which type of factors would Mr. K be able to change with rehabilitation and which ones are not modifiable?

3. Mr. K's daughter brought him to the hospital as soon as she discovered his symptoms. Describe the importance of seeking care within as soon as possible after a potential stroke.

Based on his history, it appears that Mr. K also had a trans-ischemic attack 3 months ago. Because of the concern for this patient's health, the physician immediately orders a head CT, where it is determined that he has suffered an ischemic stroke affecting the posterior inferior cerebellar artery in the brain.

4. Describe the difference between a TIA and an ischemic stroke.

5. What information would the nurse provide as part of teaching to prepare Mr. K and his daughter to undergo the head CT?

6. Explain how the nurse would educate Mr. K and his daughter about this type of stroke compared to a hemorrhagic stroke.

Following diagnosis, Mr. K is set up to receive IV recombinant tissue plasminogen activator (rtPA); the nurse is to administer a bolus dose and then Mr. K will receive the rest of the dose over the course of the next hour.

7. Explain how rtPA works to manage ischemic stroke.

8. Based on the mechanism of action, what factors would prevent Mr. K from being a candidate for receiving rtPA as treatment?

9. What signs or symptoms indicate a positive outcome that the rtPA has been effective as treatment for Mr. K's stroke?

10. What signs or symptoms would indicate that further treatment is necessary?

Rationale

An ischemic stroke occurs when an artery supplying blood to the brain is occluded, preventing certain areas of the brain from receiving oxygen and nutrients. The most common cause of ischemic stroke is atherosclerosis, however, the condition may also be caused by blood clots, drug use, or traumatic injury. A thrombotic stroke occurs when a blood clot develops in an artery in the brain and blocks the flow of blood. Alternatively, an embolic ischemic stroke occurs when a blood clot from another part of the body has broken off into circulation and traveled to the brain to lodge in one of the blood vessels.

An ischemic stroke differs from a hemorrhagic stroke in that while an ischemic stroke is caused by some type of obstruction in a vessel in the brain, a hemorrhagic stroke develops as bleeding in the brain when one of the small vessels ruptures. The patient who is experiencing a stroke may not know the difference between the two types. Once the provider knows whether the patient has had an ischemic or hemorrhagic stroke, the nurse should talk to the patient about his condition, as the types of treatment will differ between the two kinds of stroke.

There are several factors that can increase a person's risk of stroke. Modifiable risk factors include smoking, hyperlipidemia, hypertension, and lack of physical activity; non-modifiable factors include advancing age, male gender, and a family history of stroke. It is important for a person who is experiencing a stroke to receive treatment as soon as possible; each minute of waiting can cause further damage to the brain. The patient in this situation was brought in by his daughter as soon as she noticed the signs and symptoms, which is important to give him the chance to have the best possible outcome.

Some people experience a trans-ischemic attack (TIA) prior to actually having a stroke. A TIA differs from a stroke in that a TIA is a temporary condition and does not cause permanent damage as a stroke does. It may cause the same signs and symptoms of a stroke but it usually resolves within about an hour. However, up to 15 percent of patients who experience a TIA have a stroke within 3 months.

Treatment of an ischemic stroke includes administration of drugs that will break up the clot and restore circulation to the brain. If the patient started having symptoms of stroke within the last 3 hours, the most appropriate initial treatment is administration of IV recombinant tissue plasminogen activator (rtPA). rtPA works by dissolving the clot and restoring blood flow to the deprived parts of the brain. Patients who receive rtPA within 3 to 4.5 hours after suffering stroke symptoms have been shown to have improved outcomes.

rtPA is not appropriate for all stroke patients. A person who has had a hemorrhagic stroke, someone with bleeding tendencies, a person with head trauma, or someone who has recently had surgery would not be a candidate for receiving rtPA. Because rtPA dissolves the clot, it can put the stroke patient at risk of bleeding. If the patient responds favorably to the rtPA, the nurse would expect to see improvement in the patient's clinical condition and reduction of the signs and symptoms that brought him to seek care. However, if the patient does not respond, he may need further thrombolytic therapy to break up the clot or he may need surgery to try to restore blood flow to the brain.

Pneumothorax

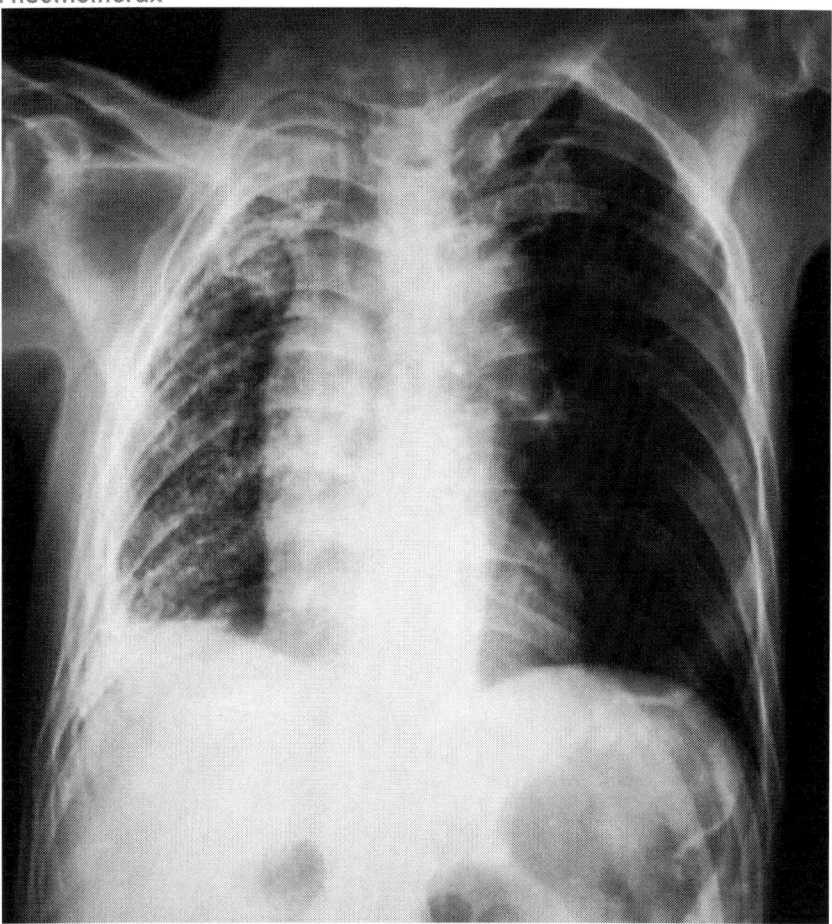

R. L is a 32-year-old male patient who is brought into the emergency department after falling from a structure at a construction site. Although he was wearing a hard had and safety vest, he fell approximately 8 feet onto a pile of lumber and landed on his right side. He remained awake after the fall and was talking to his coworkers while they called 911 and waited for help.

Emergency medical services brought the patient to the hospital. Upon arrival, R. L. is awake and alert and he has a cervical collar in place. His heart rate is elevated at 122 bpm and his respiratory rate is rapid and labored; he has an oxygen saturation of 90% on room air. He complains of pain on the right side of his chest and has notable ecchymosis and a few minor lacerations to the site. When the physician palpates the chest, the patient cries out and says he feels sharp pain.

1. Based on the information provided, outline the most appropriate nursing interventions in order to stabilize this patient.

M.L. receives a chest x-ray at the bedside, which shows a right-sided pneumothorax. Despite administration of 4 L oxygen, his saturations remain between 90 and 95%. His lung sounds are absent on the affected side, he has marked intercostal retractions, and his respiratory rate is 32/minute.

2. What is the difference between a spontaneous pneumothorax and the type that has developed in this patient's situation?

3. Since M. L. is unable to maintain adequate oxygenation, what might be the next step for improving his oxygen exchange?

4. What interventions would the nurse utilize that would promote effective airway clearance for this patient?

The physician inserts a 30F chest tube into the pleural space on the right side of the patient's chest. The nurse assists with attaching the tube to negative pressure drainage and uses a 3-chamber collection system. Following insertion, the nurse notes routine fluctuations in the water seal chamber. The patient's oxygen levels continue to fall despite the chest tube placement and the physician opts to insert an endotracheal tube and place the patient on a mechanical ventilator.

5. Which actions would the nurse perform to assist with chest tube placement?

6. What does tidaling in the water seal indicate? What does continuous bubbling in the water seal chamber indicate?

7. What signs or symptoms would the nurse monitor for that would indicate that the patient is developing complications because of his chest tube?

8. What types of assessments would the nurse need to perform to continually monitor this patient if he requires a ventilator and a chest tube?

9. What signs or symptoms would indicate that the patient's respiratory status is improving after these treatment measures?

Rationale

Commonly called a collapsed lung, a pneumothorax occurs when excess air enters the space between the visceral pleura (the membrane surrounding the lungs) and the parietal pleura (the membrane lining the interior of the lung cavity). Excess air that enters this space places extra pressure on the lung within the respiratory cavity. The lung is unable to expand as it should to facilitate appropriate gas exchange. Consequently, the lung is considered collapsed and the patient may suffer from decreased oxygenation and retained carbon dioxide. The patient in the situation described is suffering from a pneumothorax that has developed because of a traumatic event: some object or body part has punctured the space between the two pleural layers, causing the lung to collapse. Alternatively, a spontaneous pneumothorax can occur without any trauma present and may happen if the membrane becomes weakened due to some type of disease process.

When caring for a patient who has a pneumothorax, the nurse must work to improve the patient's oxygenation so that he does not become hypoxic. This means administering supplemental oxygen to keep saturation levels above ordered limits, regularly auscultating lung sounds, and monitoring the patient's respiratory patterns. A patient who develops severe respiratory compromise because of a pneumothorax may need assistance with breathing through intubation and mechanical ventilation. In many situations, a pneumothorax requires placement of a chest tube to remove the excess air and fluid in the pleural space and to allow the lung to re-expand.

Although the healthcare provider is the person who inserts the chest tube, the nurse should be available to assist. The nurse helps the patient to a comfortable position to where the provider can access the appropriate area; she also monitors the patient's hemodynamic status, provides pain medicine and sedation as ordered, educates the patient about the process, and assists with connecting the tubing to the chest tube canister once it has been inserted.

The goals of the chest tube are to remove excess air and fluid from the pleural space and to restore negative pressure so that the lung is able to re-expand. The patient may have some drainage leave the chest tube insertion site, which would be collected within the drainage unit. The unit may contain one to three chambers that collect drainage and act as a one-way valve to prevent air and fluid from entering the patient's chest. Tidaling occurs as a normal part of respiratory effort when the patient breathes in and out. The nurse can expect to see tidaling as fluctuations in the level of water in the water seal chamber while the patient breathes. The water seal chamber may also have bubbling on occasion, but if bubbling is constant, the nurse should suspect an air leak in the system.

While caring for a patient with a chest tube and a ventilator, the nurse must monitor both systems to prevent complications. Some potential complications include hypoxia, excess drainage from the chest tube site, excess drainage at the insertion site as evidenced by a saturated dressing, infection, and the collection of air in the subcutaneous tissue surrounding the insertion site. Alternatively, the patient may appear to be improving and recovering from his pneumothorax when his clinical status improves, he is hemodynamically stable, and the nurse is able to clamp the chest tube for short periods without causing further problems.

Hypertensive Crisis

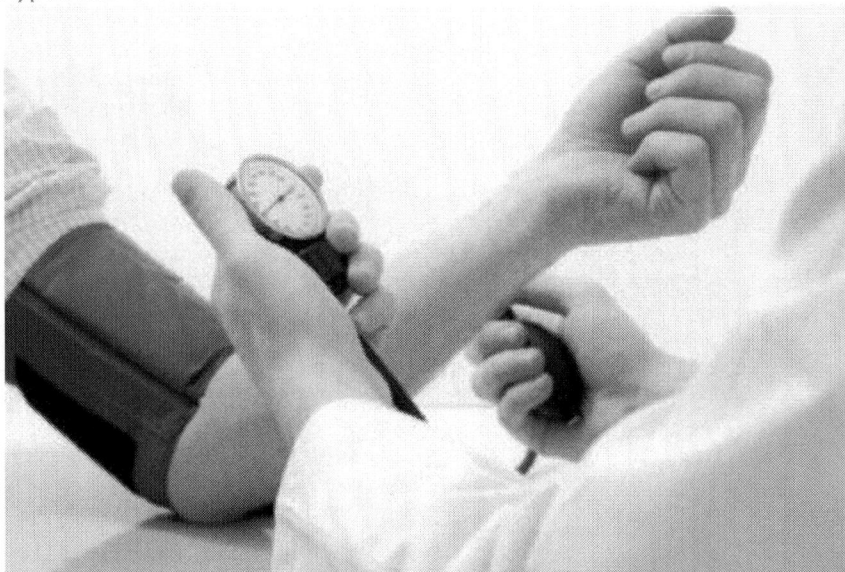

A 36-year-old pregnant patient is in the labor and delivery unit of the hospital. She is 37 weeks' gestation with her second pregnancy and has had spontaneous rupture of membranes. The patient has been followed closely by her OB/GYN because of her history of high blood pressure during both her last pregnancy and with this current pregnancy. The patient arrived in the labor and delivery unit 6 hours ago and has been having regular contractions and increasing pain and has cervical dilation of 6 cm. Upon admission to the unit, the patient's vital signs were: HR 98 bpm, RR 16/minute, BP 128/78 mmHg, T 98.1°F. The client has been taking nicardipine to control her blood pressure during this pregnancy.

The patient calls the nurse into her room because she has developed a sudden and severe headache; most of the pain is located behind her right eye. She tells the nurse that she feels dizzy and asks her to turn off the overhead light because she says it hurts her eyes. The nurse performs a rapid assessment and notes that the patient's HR is 116 bpm and her pulse is full and bounding; her BP is 168/120 mmHg and she is breathing rapidly.

1. The nurse suspects that the patient is experiencing a hypertensive crisis as a result of pre-eclampsia and based on her symptoms and her blood pressure. What other signs or symptoms would be present for this patient to be diagnosed as having a hypertensive emergency?

2. What potential body system complications could develop as a result of unresolved hypertensive crisis?

The nurse performs a rapid urinalysis test from a sample of the patient's urine, which demonstrates elevated levels of urinary protein. After contacting the physician, the nurse receives orders to check a complete metabolic panel and to get an ECG stat. The nurse checks the fetal monitor to ensure that the baby is not in distress because of the mother's condition.

3. After completing the physician's orders, describe in order the interventions the nurse would perform to control this patient's condition.

4. What changes in laboratory levels would the nurse expect to see in a patient with hypertensive crisis?

5. Explain why a patient might have elevated protein levels in the urine when experiencing a hypertensive crisis.

The nurse reports the laboratory results to the physician and then receives orders to administer labetolol IV 20 mg bolus and then 2mg/min continuously. The nurse is also to check BP levels every 5 minutes and notify the provider if the diastolic BP remains over 100 mmHg after 20 minutes. The physician is coming to the hospital to check the patient's delivery status and the nurse prepares to assist with an emergent delivery if necessary.

6. What side effects should the nurse monitor for when administering labetolol?

7. If the medication begins to work as it should, what type of patient response would the nurse expect to see?

Rationale

Hypertensive crisis describes a situation in which a patient experiences very high blood pressure that causes organ damage. The signs or symptoms the patient experiences are often related to the organ damage present and the cause of the condition. For example, a patient who has altered kidney function as a result of hypertensive crisis would demonstrate not only high blood pressure, but possibly changes in electrolyte levels or decreased urinary output.

Unresolved hypertensive crisis can lead to significant complications, including hemorrhage from ruptured blood vessels, heart failure, and kidney damage, and ultimately, death. In this situation, both the mother and the baby are at risk of injury or death from hypertensive crisis. If the nurse determines that the patient is experiencing hypertensive crisis, she should contact the physician right away; she may need to provide oxygen, elevate the head of the bed, and give medications that can decrease the patient's blood pressure. The nurse caring for this patient would also need to continue to monitor fetal heart patterns to ensure that the baby is not being negatively affected.

Because hypertensive crisis causes such high blood pressure and organ dysfunction, the physician may order some laboratory tests that would check to see what areas of dysfunction are present. These tests may include urinalysis, a metabolic profile, ECG, chest x-ray, or head CT. Again, the type of test administered depends on the target organ suspected of dysfunction. In this situation, the patient has elevated protein levels in the urine, and the nurse suspects kidney damage. The patient would have elevated protein in the urine if the kidneys are not functioning well, since the kidneys are responsible for filtering substances such as protein in the bloodstream. The nurse should assess for other signs of kidney damage, including changes in urine output or an altered level of consciousness in the patient.

Treatment of hypertensive crisis requires close monitoring by the nurse, with possible admission to the ICU. A patient in labor and delivery must be monitored very closely through delivery and then may need to be transferred to ICU after the baby is born. The goal of treatment is to get the patient's blood pressure into a normal range with as few of complications as possible. This typically involves administration of IV medications such as labetolol or nicardipine, which act as vasodilators to increase the size of blood vessels and reduce blood pressure levels. These drugs are short acting and will control hypertension, however, they do not necessarily cause a rapid drop in blood pressure. Instead, the nurse should expect that the patient's blood pressure would more likely come down slowly to a stable level. If the patient's blood pressure continues to be problematic, the nurse may need to prepare for rapid delivery of the infant, such as through cesarean section, to protect both the mother and the baby.

End-Stage Renal Disease (ESRD)

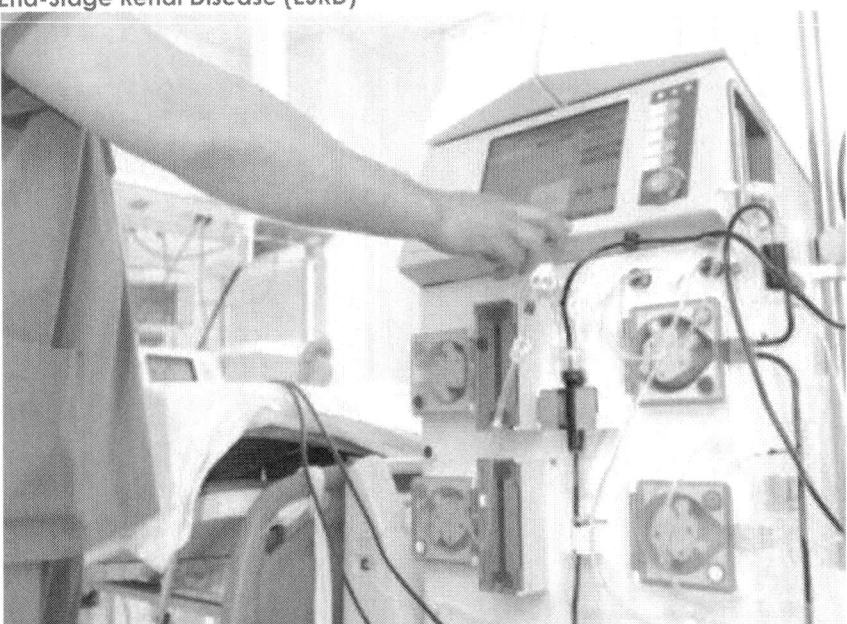

R. G. is a 61-year-old female patient who is being seen as part of ongoing care. During her assessment, she tells the nurse that she has been feeling much worse over the course of the past 2 weeks. Her skin is very dry and itchy, she has headaches, and she complains of feeling exhausted. R. G. was diagnosed with type 2 diabetes 8 years ago and has developed chronic kidney disease, in which she takes diuretic medications and has a modified diabetic diet that is low in protein. Her last GFR was checked 1 month ago and was 28 mL/min/1.73m^2.

The physician orders lab work and diagnostic testing. Her lab results are as follows: Hgb: 3.8/mcl, Platelets: 100,000/mcL, BUN: 32 mg/dL, Cr: 3.8 mg/dL, Na: 131 mEq/L, K: 3.7 mEq/L, Glucose: 166 mg/dL. Her urinalysis shows that she has excess protein and glucose in the urine. Her GFR is 14 mL/min/1.73m^2. The nurse notes that R. G. seems very fatigued and appears disoriented at times throughout the assessment.

1. Describe how chronic renal failure differs from acute renal failure.

2. At what point is a person with chronic renal failure considered to be in end-stage renal disease?

Based on R. G.'s lab results and symptoms, the physician has determined that the patient's kidney disease has progressed and she now is in a state of end-stage renal disease (ESRD). The nurse receives the following orders for medications to give to the patient:

Epogen 100 units/kg SQ
Periactin 4 mg PO tid

3. Describe why these drugs would be ordered for R. G.'s condition.

4. What signs or symptoms would the nurse expect to see that would indicate that these medications are working?

Following administration of the medications, the nurse receives further orders to prepare R. G. for hemodialysis. The patient has not undergone dialysis in the past and she does not have an access port for the procedure. She is scheduled for placement of a vascular access device and then will receive her first round of dialysis in her hospital room upon return.

5. What information should the nurse include as part of teaching about the vascular access device and dialysis?

6. Explain how a vascular access device works to use for dialysis.

7. Describe the basic process of hemodialysis.

R. G. has returned from the cath lab with a vascular access device in place and is started on hemodialysis. Her first treatment takes place in her hospital room with a portable machine but she will later need ongoing dialysis when her condition stabilizes. The nurse reviews information with the patient about lifestyle changes and self-care now that she has ESRD.

8. Explain what medications the patient would most likely need on a routine basis now that she will need regular hemodialysis.

9. What are the patient's options for receiving hemodialysis once her condition stabilizes?

10. Review the important information the nurse should provide to this patient about placement and care of a vascular access device.

11. What follow-up tests would be necessary to ensure that the hemodialysis is working?

Rationale

Chronic kidney disease describes the gradual loss of kidney function that occurs after damage. It differs from acute kidney disease in that it takes much longer and has a gradual onset, whereas acute kidney disease may occur from an illness or infection and the patient suffers the effects right away. The final stage of chronic kidney disease is end-stage renal disease (ESRD), in which the patient's kidney function is so poor that dialysis is required. The patient may have glomerular function checked to determine kidney function; ESRD is considered when a person's glomerular filtration rate (GFR) is less than 15 mL/min/1.73m^2.

A patient with ESRD will have changes in the blood cells and with electrolyte levels in the bloodstream, since the kidneys are not working effectively. The kidneys normally produce erythropoietin, which stimulate the body to produce red blood cells. A patient with ESRD may then have fewer red blood cells and would require medications that would supplement erythropoietin; in some cases, the patient may also need a blood transfusion. Persons with ESRD also suffer from a number of other physical symptoms, including dry, itchy skin as a result of electrolyte abnormalities. In this situation, Periactin is prescribed to help control some of the itching this patient is experiencing.

ESRD requires hemodialysis and if the patient is a candidate, kidney transplant. This patient's kidney function has continued to decline and she will die if she does not have dialysis. The patient needs a vascular access device, such as an arteriovenous (AV) fistula or graft. This type of device connects the artery and vein together so that the dialysis machine can remove blood and then return it to the same site. During hemodialysis, blood is removed and run through the dialysis machine that has a filter known as a dialyzer. The filter removes excess fluid and waste products and then returns the blood back to the patient.

Most patients need to have hemodialysis about 3 times per week. The majority of those who receive hemodialysis do so at a clinic designed to provide dialysis for people in the community. It takes several hours each time and normally, the patients attend their sessions and then return later in the week to repeat the process. Hemodialysis may also be performed at home for some patients. In certain situations, a person may have hemodialysis at home by connecting to the machine at night and going through the process while sleeping. This may be an option that the patient in the example could have as part of treatment.

The patient in this case would most likely have questions about her condition and about starting dialysis. The nurse should be available to provide answers as needed. The patient will also need education about diet, as she may have dietary restrictions, particularly with her diabetes and advanced stage of renal disease. It will also help to discuss the patient's prognosis and options to improve her quality of life while undergoing dialysis.

Cirrhosis

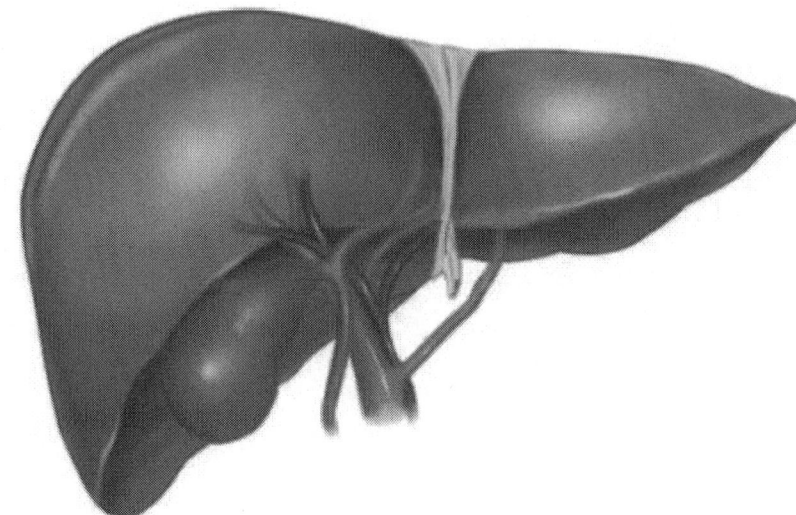

A nurse is working on the medical-surgical unit of the hospital and is starting her shift for the day. One of her patient's, Mr. W, is in the hospital for exacerbation of symptoms related to cirrhosis. Mr. W is a 55-year-old patient who has a history of alcohol use disorder, having abused alcohol for 33 years; he also suffers from atrial fibrillation and gastroesophageal reflux disease, and he is a smoker. He was admitted to the hospital last evening for abdominal pain.

Upon assessment, the nurse notes that Mr. W has pale skin with a slightly yellowish hue; his abdomen is full and rounded and he has 3+ pitting edema in the ankles bilaterally. He complains that his skin feels itchy and he is very tired. He rates his abdominal pain as a "6" on a scale of 1 to 10.

1. Mr. W's condition is caused by his history of alcohol abuse. Explain how chronic alcohol abuse causes cirrhosis of the liver.

2. List other potential causes of cirrhosis that are unrelated to alcohol intake.

3. What type of diagnostic tests would Mr. W have had that would have confirmed his diagnosis of cirrhosis?

4. What activities or lifestyle factors would most likely worsen Mr. W's condition?

Mr. W undergoes an ultrasound, which confirms that he has abdominal ascites. The nurse sets up and prepares to assist the physician with paracentesis to remove the excess fluid from Mr. W's abdomen.

5. Describe the process of performing a paracentesis to control ascites.

6. What is the nurse's role while assisting with this procedure?

7. What signs or symptoms from Mr. W would indicate complications as a result of the paracentesis?

Mr. W. tolerates the paracentesis well and the nurse administers midazolam for sedation. The physician has ordered that Mr. W rest and he is placed on NPO status with an order for TPN to support his nutritional intake. He is to receive a dose of spironolactone and to have a metabolic panel to check his electrolyte levels.

8. What electrolyte imbalances would the nurse most likely expect to see with Mr. W's condition?

9. Explain why Mr. W has been placed NPO and he is receiving parenteral nutrition.

10. What types of complications would the nurse need to monitor for while Mr. W receives TPN?

11. The nurse has given Mr. W a nursing diagnosis of Fluid Volume Excess related to his ascites and peripheral edema. What interventions would be most appropriate with this nursing diagnosis?

12. List 3 other potential nursing diagnoses that would be appropriate for Mr. W.

Rationale

Cirrhosis is a form of chronic liver disease that occurs when liver cells are destroyed and then replaced by fibrotic tissue. This tissue does not function in the same manner as normal liver tissue and consequently, the liver is unable to perform its normal functions. The most common cause of cirrhosis is chronic alcohol use, but it could also develop because of malnutrition, infection, or intake of toxic substances, such as with a medication overdose. Cirrhosis is often diagnosed based on the patient's history and physical exam, as well as other laboratory tests that confirm that the liver is not working properly. Some blood tests may check bilirubin levels, clotting factors, and liver enzymes, which would all be affected by cirrhosis. Cirrhosis can cause ascites, which is accumulation of fluid in the abdominal cavity. The patient may have such a large accumulation of fluid that it is difficult for him to breathe adequately.

A paracentesis is performed to remove the abdominal fluid that builds up to cause ascites. It is typically done at the bedside in the hospital by a healthcare provider, but the nurse will need to assist with the procedure. The paracentesis should temporarily remove the excess fluid that has built up in the abdomen because of cirrhosis. During a paracentesis, the patient lies on his back and the provider inserts a needle into the abdominal cavity after applying a local anesthetic to the site. The needle is connected to a small tube that drains the fluid and collects it in a container. The nurse should assist with the paracentesis by helping to set up the equipment for the physician and educating the patient about the procedure. During the paracentesis, the nurse should watch the patient's vital signs and help with collection of lab specimens taken of the fluid. Afterward, the nurse must monitor the injection site and check the amount of fluid that has been removed. The nurse would also ensure that no more fluid leaks from the site and that the patient does not have excess bleeding.

The patient in the example is at risk of some complications as part of undergoing paracentesis, including bleeding, hypotension, and infection at the insertion site. The patient is also at risk of electrolyte imbalance and poor nutrition because of his condition. The nurse should monitor electrolyte levels such as sodium and potassium, as well as other values such as glucose, ammonia, and protein in the blood and urine. The nurse may also need to administer enteral or parenteral nutrition to ensure that the patient gets enough vitamins and nutrients. In this case, the patient has been placed on NPO status to allow for GI rest and to reduce the stress on the liver. If the nurse administers TPN to maintain the patient's nutrition status, she would need to continue to monitor for signs of infection, hyperglycemia, and electrolyte imbalances, which are common complications associated with TPN.

This patient also has fluid volume excess as a result of liver damage and ascites. In some cases, a client will be given diuretic medications to continue to excrete fluid through the urine. The nurse should check for recurring ascites or peripheral edema and assess breath sounds to ensure that the patient is able to breathe adequately. Other possible nursing diagnoses for this condition might include Imbalanced Nutrition, Impaired Skin Integrity, Ineffective Breathing Pattern, and Risk for Injury.

Acute MI (STEMI)

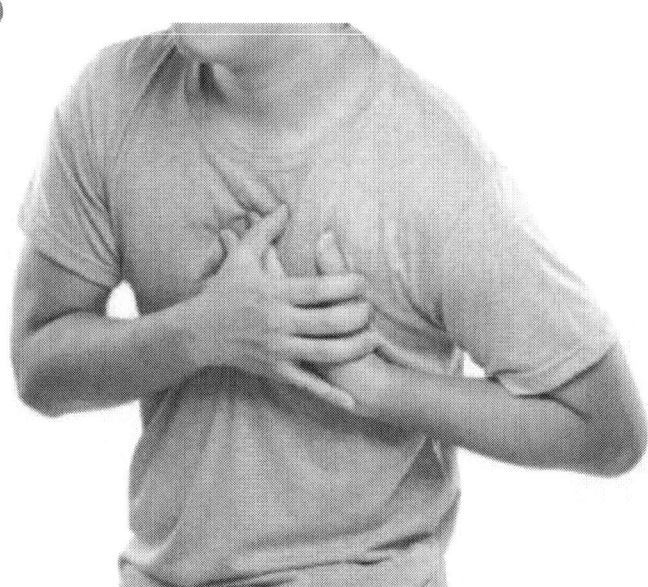

Mr. M. is a 50-year-old male patient who came in to the emergency department with complaints of chest pain while mowing his lawn. He is accompanied by his wife, who says that he was working in the yard and had to call for help because of his discomfort. He complains of chest pain, rated at a "7" on a 0 to 10 scale and describes it as a feeling of pressure in the center of his chest. The pain does not radiate to any other location. He has nausea that developed 2 hours ago and he vomited once. Upon exam, he is breathing rapidly and is diaphoretic and he appears anxious. Mr. M tells the nurse, "I think I am having a heart attack."

The patient has a history of hyperlipidemia, in which he takes atorvastatin, and hypertension, in which he takes nifedipine. He does not have a history of angina and has never experienced chest pain; because of this, he is concerned that he has not had any warning signals prior to this event. He started smoking cigarettes in high school and smoked about 1 pack per day for 18 years before successfully quitting.

1. How should the nurse explain the relationship between a patient's lack of history of angina and an acute MI?

2. Describe the factors that would determine the severity of this patient's MI.

Mr. M has an ECG and has several blood tests to check cardiac enzymes, including creatine kinase, troponin, and myoglobin levels. The ECG shows an anterior wall ST elevation myocardial infarction (STEMI).

3. Explain the difference between a STEMI and a NSTEMI and how these two conditions would be treated.

4. What nursing interventions would the nurse employ first after learning of the diagnosis of a STEMI?

5. Describe the changes in cardiac enzymes that would most likely develop because this patient is having an MI.

6. Based on the fact that the patient has a STEMI as seen on ECG, would the physician wait to find out the cardiac enzyme results before providing treatment? Why or why not?

The nurse gives Mr. M a dose of nitroglycerin and prepares him for PCI. After administration of the drug, Mr. M states that his pain level has dropped to a "3" on a 0 to 10 scale.

7. Describe how PCI would be used to manage this patient's condition.

8. What information would the nurse give to this patient that would best teach him about what to expect when receiving PCI?

9. Explain the nurse's role while in care of a patient undergoing PCI.

Rationale

An acute myocardial infarction (MI), also known as a heart attack, occurs when the heart muscle experiences ischemia and eventual necrosis of tissue as a result of lack of blood flow. This usually occurs because of some form of occlusion in the coronary blood vessels that supply blood to the heart muscle. The severity of an MI depends on the amount of occlusion in the artery, how long the occlusion has been present, and whether other vessels nearby are also occluded. Some factors increase the risk of a person having an MI, including a history of hyperlipidemia or diabetes, male gender, history of hypertension, family history of MI, and tobacco use. The patient in this example suffers from hyperlipidemia and he is a male; additionally, he has a smoking history even though he currently does not smoke tobacco. Angina may occur in some cases before an MI; angina is chest pain and pressure that may feel like a heart attack and it develops because of decreased oxygen reaching the heart muscle. Approximately 50 percent of people who suffer an MI will have a history of angina.

An MI may be classified as a STEMI or an NSTEMI, depending on the outcome of the ECG. A STEMI (myocardial infarction marked by S-T elevation) will demonstrate changes in the S-T segment on the ECG; it typically occurs with a complete occlusion of a coronary artery after the rupture of plaque from atherosclerosis. Alternatively, a NSTEMI may indicate an incomplete occlusion and there is still a small amount of blood flow through the artery.

A STEMI is a medical emergency, and the nurse must know how to rapidly respond in this situation. The nurse may need to administer medications as ordered, including nitroglycerin or aspirin, as well as continue to manage the patient's airway, breathing efforts, and hemodynamic status, with particular assessment of cardiac arrhythmias. The physician may order lab testing, such as for cardiac enzymes, to determine the extent of damage. Although cardiac enzymes may be helpful in assessing the situation, the provider may not wait to determine their results before advancing to treatment of a STEMI. This is because the condition requires such rapid intervention that if a STEMI has been recognized, the patient should be treated as soon as possible without waiting for these types of lab results.

The main treatment of a STEMI is percutaneous coronary intervention (PCI), which should be performed within 90 minutes of arrival at the hospital. PCI involves taking the patient to the cardiac cath lab and performing percutaneous coronary angioplasty (PTCA), in which dye is injected into the patient's circulation through a femoral catheter and the physician can identify the location of the blockage. A balloon-tipped catheter is then inserted into the site of the occlusion and inflated to open the blood vessel. The physician may also place a stent at the site that will keep the vessel open.

The goal of PCI is to restore blood flow to the heart. Following the procedure, the patient will need to remain on bedrest for a prescribed period. The nurse's role is to monitor the patient's hemodynamic status and ensure that his cardiac function is improving. The patient is at risk of bleeding from the catheter insertion site and the nurse must ensure that the patient does not move the affected leg, that he stays on bedrest, and that the site is intact.

Hypothyroidism

L. R. is a 35-year-old female patient who is being seen for a post-op exam following a partial thyroidectomy 1 month ago. The patient had developed a benign nodule on her thyroid that continued to grow and was starting to affect her swallowing abilities. She underwent a partial thyroidectomy 4 weeks ago and had an uncomplicated recovery. At the follow-up exam, L. R. complains of feeling extremely tired and says that she never was able to return to the same state of activity she had before her surgery. Sometimes, she has difficulty getting out of bed. She has gained 5 lbs. since her surgery and she complains of feeling cold all the time. She often has muscle aches and joint pain, for which she takes acetaminophen for pain relief. Her vital signs are HR 60 bpm, RR 12/minute, BP 110/70 mmHg, and T 98.0°F.

1. The patient is most likely suffering from hypothyroidism as a result of her thyroidectomy. Explain how removal of part of the thyroid gland would cause the patient's symptoms.

2. Describe the major roles of T3, T4, and TSH in the body.

The physician gives orders for L. R. to have a TSH level drawn at the lab and the results are 8.6 mIU/L. The physician then orders levothyroxine 75mcg po daily because of the patient's thyroid hormone levels. The nurse gives the client a prescription for the medication and provides teaching about what to expect when taking it.

3. How does levothyroxine work in the treatment of hypothyroidism?

4. What signs or symptoms should the nurse tell the client to look for that would be side effects of using levothyroxine?

5. Does the patient need to take this medication every day? Why or why not?

The nurse sets up an appointment for L.R. to return to the clinic in one month after she has had a chance to take the medication and to recheck her thyroid hormone levels. The patient is also instructed about the complications of untreated hypothyroidism.

6. What types of complications could this patient develop if she does not take her thyroid supplement?

7. What is myxedema? How does this condition develop as a result of untreated hypothyroidism?

8. What is a goiter? How would a goiter be treated if the patient were to develop this condition?

Rationale

Hypothyroidism describes a condition in which the thyroid is underactive and does not produce enough thyroid hormone to meet the body's needs. Deficiency of thyroid hormone can cause a variety of symptoms that range from mild to severe. Thyroid function can be checked by laboratory tests that measure some of the main types of thyroid hormones. Thyroid-stimulating hormone (TSH) stimulates the thyroid gland to create hormones. Activation of TSH starts in the hypothalamus of the brain. When TSH levels are high, the person is said to have hypothyroidism because the body is trying to stimulate the thyroid gland to produce more thyroid hormones. A TSH level is one of the main laboratory tests used to detect hypothyroidism. T3, also called triiodothyronine, and T4, called thyroxine, are important for upholding the body's metabolism and are part of the work of most body systems, including the heart, GI tract, the muscles, and the brain.

When the patient has hypothyroidism, she will need supplemental thyroid hormone. Most patients, when diagnosed with hypothyroidism because of a surgical condition, such as in the case example, will need to take thyroid supplements for life. Thyroid supplement medication is available as a synthetic substitute in a tablet that can be taken daily. The most common type of thyroid supplement is levothyroxine (Synthroid), although there are many other types of supplements as well, including some natural thyroid supplements that come from porcine samples.

When a person starts taking levothyroxine, the nurse needs to educate her about the importance of taking the drug as prescribed, as failing to take the supplement routinely can cause thyroid hormone levels to drop. The patient needs to continue to take the medication because it acts as a supplement and fills in for the abnormal thyroid hormones. The nurse needs to educate the patient about the potential side effects she may experience with levothyroxine; some side effects include weight changes and high blood pressure. Because levothyroxine is a thyroid hormone supplement that affects so many different body systems, the patient may have a number of side effects, including cardiac arrhythmias, skin inflammation, and mood changes.

Untreated hypothyroidism can cause significant complications. In this situation, because part of the patient's thyroid gland has been removed, the remaining gland may attempt to produce more thyroid hormone to keep up with the demands of the body. Without supplementation, the remaining thyroid gland may eventually exhaust its ability to maintain enough thyroid hormone. Myxedema is a potential complication of untreated hypothyroidism; it occurs as changes in a person's level of consciousness that eventually leads to coma and death if it is not managed. Myxedema develops because the levels of thyroid hormone available are so low that the person lapses into a coma. A goiter is another type of complication that could develop with untreated hypothyroidism. A goiter is a growth of the thyroid gland that occurs when the body tries to make up for low levels of thyroid hormone. The brain stimulates the thyroid gland to try and produce more thyroid hormone and the gland starts to grow in size. The nurse's main role in caring for a patient with hypothyroidism is education about the condition. Because it can cause so many different symptoms and complications, hypothyroidism requires extensive teaching about how the patient can best care for herself.

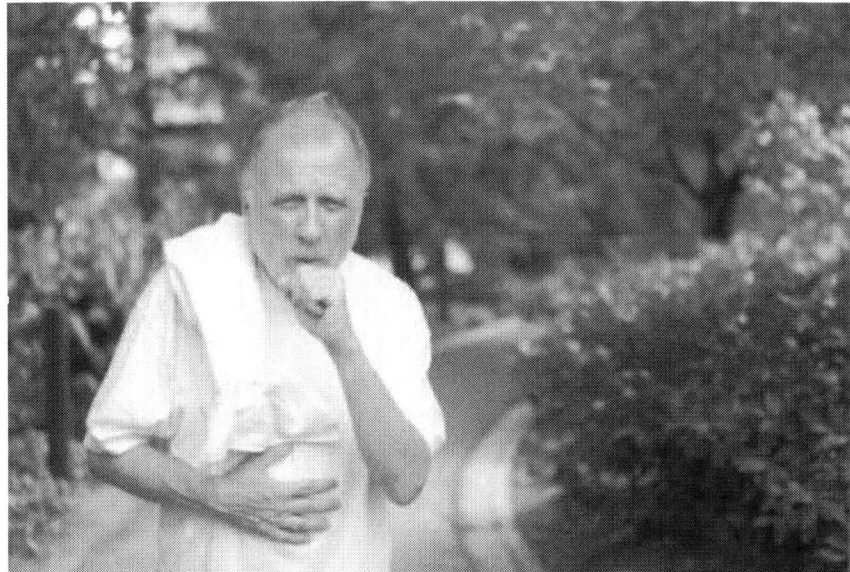

J. D. is a 68-year-old male patient who is in the hospital for assessment and treatment of increased difficulties with breathing. J. D. is a lifelong 2 ppd smoker, starting when he was 15 years old and continuing to the present time. He was diagnosed with emphysema 3 years ago and uses supplemental oxygen in the home.

J. D. was admitted to the hospital from his doctor's office where he was having a physical exam done by the nurse practitioner. He presented for his check-up with acute shortness of breath as well as substernal and intercostal retractions. His respiratory rate is 24/minute and his oxygen saturations are 90% on 3L of O2 by nasal prongs. He stated at his exam that he has had increasingly more difficulties with breathing and performing activities of daily living, becoming short of breath with activities such as eating or talking, when he was not having a problem before. After admission to the hospital, the nurse helps J. D. to his bed with the head of it elevated; his oxygen amount is increased to 6 L per nasal prongs, and the nurse is awaiting further orders from the physician.

1. Explain the pathologic changes that occur in lung tissue when a person develops emphysema.

2. List risk factors that are most commonly associated with development of chronic obstructive pulmonary disease.

3. Explain how the nurse would teach J. D. about using oxygen at home and continuing to smoke.

J. D.'s physician has ordered spirometry testing, which indicates that the patient's severity of COPD is stage II. He is given a prescription for inhaled corticosteroids, and the nurse explains how to use the medication for his condition, demonstrating how to use it the first time.

4. What does a classification of stage II COPD indicate?

5. Describe how corticosteroids would work to treat this patient's condition.

6. What other drugs might J. D. be prescribed to control his COPD symptoms?

7. Would the physician prescribe antibiotics in this case? Why or why not?

Rationale

Chronic obstructive pulmonary disease (COPD) is a chronic and progressive lung disease that affects the size of the airways and the ability of the alveoli to perform adequate gas exchange. COPD is usually classified as either chronic bronchitis or emphysema. A person with emphysema has stretching and rupture of the alveoli in the lungs so that they do not work properly. The person becomes short of breath and has decreased levels of oxygen in the bloodstream because of the damaged alveoli. The most common cause of COPD is smoking, although there are other factors that contribute as well, such as chronic exposure to environmental allergens, or alpha-1 anti-trypsin deficiency, which is a genetic lack of an enzyme that protects the lung tissue. The patient in this example is at risk of injury, not only because of his lung disease, but also because he continues to smoke while using oxygen. Oxygen is not a flammable substance, but it is required to support a flame. If the person had even a small flame or spark nearby while using oxygen, such as when smoking, the oxygen could cause the fire to rampantly burn out of control. The nurse must educate this patient about the dangers of continuing to smoke while using supplemental oxygen.

There is no cure for COPD and because it is a progressive disease, the patient's condition can be expected to worsen. This is particularly true when a patient continues to smoke after diagnosis. Diagnosis of the condition is done after taking the patient's history and performing a physical exam; the patient may undergo testing through spirometry to determine if there is obstruction present that is causing respiratory difficulties. Once diagnosed, the patient may later be checked to determine the level of severity, as classified through a staging system. The severity of COPD is measured by assessment of forced expiratory volume in 1 second (FEV_1) as measured through spirometry. A classification of stage II COPD indicates moderately severe disease.

There are several medications that could be administered to help the patient with his COPD symptoms. Although these drugs do not cure the condition, they can make it more tolerable for the patient to live with COPD. Drugs such as bronchodilators, which work by increasing the size of the airways, are commonly prescribed for symptom control. Additionally, corticosteroids reduce the amount of swelling and inflammation in the airway that could contribute to further scarring. The patient in this situation would not need antibiotics, as he is not suffering from an infection because of his symptoms; antibiotics would be useless in treating the symptoms of this patient's COPD.

Because COPD is a chronic illness, management is focused on short-term control of breathing issues and exacerbations of the illness. The patient would most likely benefit from pulmonary rehabilitation, which can help him with lifestyle changes needed to modify his activity levels and to improve his quality of life while living with this progressive illness.

Seizure Disorder

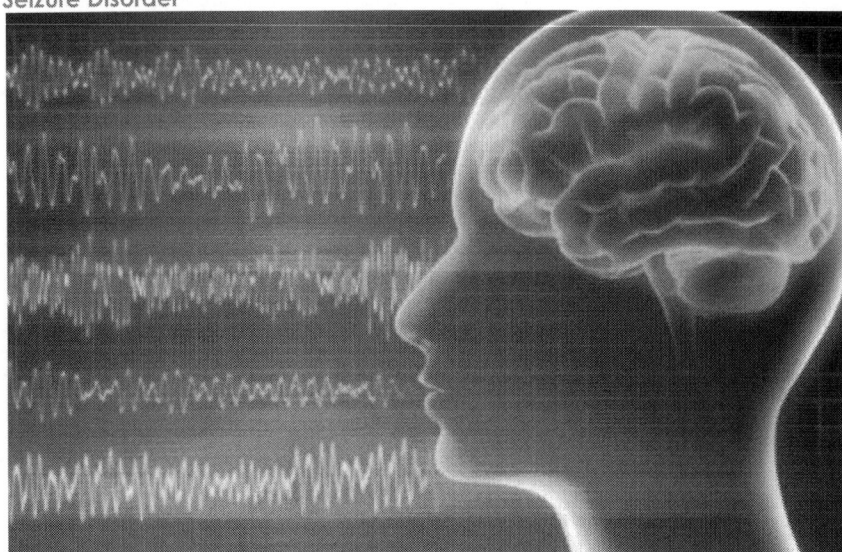

A nurse is caring for a 7-year-old child in the primary care clinic who has come to the office for a routine physical exam for school. As an infant, the patient developed meningitis and was hospitalized; she developed a seizure disorder as a result of the condition and has a tonic-clonic seizure approximately once every 3 months, despite taking prescribed anticonvulsant medications.

During the visit, the patient's mother tells the nurse that the patient had a seizure last night; it had been 4 months since the child's last seizure. She has been active in school and is in the 1st grade, she is part of an afterschool program, and she plays sports. However, she has been experiencing more stress recently because her father was injured at work and has been home recovering from his injuries. The patient's mother worries that she will continue to have more seizures because of her stress levels.

1. What is the difference between a person who experiences a seizure and someone who has a seizure disorder (epilepsy)?

2. Describe the difference between tonic-clonic, myoclonic, generalized, and absence seizures.

The nurse continues to talk to the mother about triggers in the child's life that may contribute to seizures. The child is otherwise in good physical health and was not injured during the seizure; however, the nurse would like to discuss the patient's emotional state a little further to determine if there are other psychological issues affecting the patient's condition.

3. What types of triggers might be present that could cause a person with a seizure disorder to experience a seizure?

4. How would the nurse educate this mother about controlling triggers in her child's life to reduce the risk of seizure activity?

5. What information should the nurse present about how to keep the patient safe during a seizure?

The nurse reviews the patient's anticonvulsant medications with her mother. The child has been prescribed phenobarbital 85 mg daily to control seizure activity. After discussing the child's condition with the physician, it is determined that the dose of phenobarbital should be increased to 100 mg daily in order to better control seizure activity.

6. What types of side effects would the nurse expect to see in a child who is using this phenobarbital?

7. Describe the possible effects the family can expect to see in the child after the dose of phenobarbital has increased.

The nurse has given the child a nursing diagnosis of Risk for Injury related to her seizure activity and provides the family with a seizure action plan for what to do if the child has another seizure at home or if away from home, such as while at school or camp.

8. What types of nursing interventions are most appropriate with a Risk for Injury diagnosis in this patient?

9. List three potential outcomes that would be expected of this patient after implementing interventions with this nursing diagnosis.

Rationale

A person with a seizure disorder is someone who has had at least 2 seizures that have occurred at least 24 hours apart. The condition is also called epilepsy. When seizures occur in someone with a seizure disorder, they can be classified as being one of various types; some types include tonic-clonic (grand mal), myoclonic, generalized, or absence (petit mal) seizures. Tonic-clonic seizures are some of the most well-known; they are also frightening to those witnessing the event. During a tonic-clonic seizure, a person loses consciousness and the muscles become rigid; after a few moments, the muscles begin to spasm and the body jerks uncontrollably.

A myoclonic seizure occurs when a person experiences a short contraction of muscles; the situation has been described as being similar to a shock or jolt. The seizure often lasts for a very brief time but it can be dangerous if it occurs while a person is engaging in certain activities. Generalized seizures are those that can start from any point in the brain; the exact point of onset of a generalized seizure is often unknown. This compares with a partial seizure, which seems to start at one area of the brain and that may or may not affect a person's level of consciousness. Absence (petit mal) seizures occur as a disturbance in brain function but the person does not typically exhibit muscle spasms. Instead, a person having an absence seizure may stare blankly, stop talking, or make facial movements.

People who have seizure disorders may have triggers in their lives that increase the risk of having a seizure. Triggers are often environmental stimuli; some common triggers described by people with seizure disorders include stress, changes in temperature, bright light, spicy food, alcohol or caffeine intake, and fatigue. When a person has a diagnosed seizure disorder, it is important to recognize the factors that may be triggers to seizures and try to control those triggers. In the situation described, the child may have experienced a seizure because she was feeling stress about her father's health. The nurse can talk with the child's mother about seizure triggers and the best ways to control them.

A patient with a seizure disorder is at risk of being injured during the seizure, particularly if she is performing some type of activity that could cause her to get hurt. A person having a tonic-clonic seizure will usually fall down and lose consciousness, which can be very dangerous. While providing direct care of a patient having a seizure, the nurse should take measures to keep her safe, such as by moving sharp objects away from the patient or putting a pillow under the head. The nurse should never try to put something in the patient's mouth, even though there are stories of people being injured by clenching their jaws or swallowing the tongue. Most people just need some room and need to be protected from injury during a seizure.

Phenobarbital is one of the most common types of anticonvulsants prescribed for management of seizures. It can be used in children but it can also cause drowsiness and in some cases, it may lead to hyperactivity. The parent of a child who takes this drug should monitor for changes in the child's level of consciousness and her activity levels, particularly if the dose is changed. With the increase in the amount of phenobarbital, it can be expected that the child may have behavior changes but could also have a decrease in seizure activity as well.

Sepsis

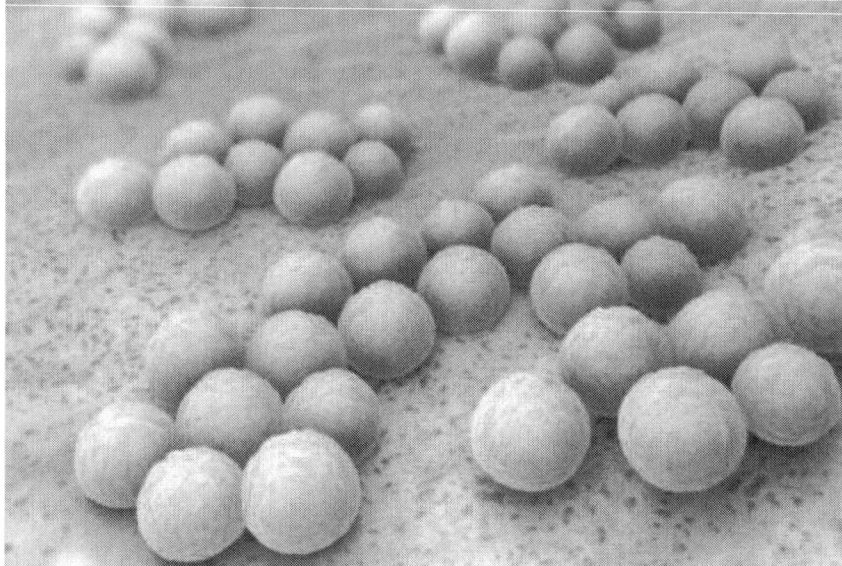

M. C. is a 71-year-old male patient who has been admitted to the hospital for complaints of abdominal pain and fever. M. C. was diagnosed with chronic myelogenous leukemia last year and receives a round of chemotherapy approximately once per month. His other medical history includes mild hypothyroidism and gastroesophageal reflux disease.

Upon admission, M. C. complains of right upper quadrant pain rated as an "8" on a 0 to 10 scale. He has significant tenderness with palpation and his abdomen is guarded. His temperature is 101.9°F and he is alert and oriented. He is accompanied by his wife and daughter. Further diagnostic testing through an abdominal CT reveals that M. C. has a severely inflamed gall bladder with the presence of a number of small stones in the common bile duct. M. C. is scheduled to undergo a laparoscopic cholescytectomy that same day.

Prior to his surgery, the nurse inserts an indwelling catheter and administers 2g of ampicillin IV as a prophylactic antibiotic as ordered by the physician. M. C. continues to wait in his hospital room for the time when he will go to surgery. The nurse notes through his routine vital sign checks that M. C.'s blood pressure is dropping and he appears listless.

1. After the nurse notes these signs and symptoms from M. C., what actions should the nurse should perform next?

2. Describe how this patient's condition puts him at higher risk of complications associated with his surgery.

The nurse contacts the physician about M. C.'s status; the physician orders that the patient be placed on continuous hemodynamic monitoring with blood pressure checks every 5 minutes. The physician has also ordered several lab tests, including a CBC, blood glucose, and blood culture. The results of the blood tests are as follows: WBC: 2,800 cells/mcL, RBC: 4.0/mcL, platelets: 55,000/mcL, Hgb: 10.2 g/dL, Hct: 35.8%, glucose: 167 mg/dL. The blood culture is pending.

3. Describe the difference between systemic inflammatory response syndrome (SIRS) and sepsis.

4. Explain why M. C. most likely has these lab results.

5. Based on the results of these lab tests, which action of the nurse would be most important?

The nurse receives an order to administer 2 units of fresh frozen plasma and M. C. is taken back to surgery before waiting any longer. Following the cholecystectomy, M. C. is intubated and sedated, but he is having a difficult time waking up. His vital signs are as follows: HR 108 bpm, RR 16/minute (on a timed cycle of the ventilator) BP 86/50 mmHg, T: 100.9°F. He is taken to the ICU where he is cared for on a ventilator and placed on a hemodynamic monitor. The physician inserts a Swan-Ganz catheter to monitor internal blood pressure and also orders levophed to be added to the IV. The nurse continues to closely monitor M.C.'s condition and is assigned as a 1:1 nurse-to-patient ratio because of his condition.

6. What is the purpose of administering levophed IV?

7. Why would the nurse administer fresh frozen plasma to this patient before surgery?

8. What type of complications is M. C. at risk of?

9. Describe the purpose of a Swan-Ganz catheter and why it would be most useful in this situation.

Rationale

Sepsis is a condition that occurs in almost 1 million people each year; it is caused by widespread infection from bacteria, fungi, a virus, or a parasite. A patient with sepsis may be experiencing systemic inflammatory response syndrome (SIRS), which is indicated by an elevated temperature, tachycardia, tachypnea, and either an increased or decreased WBC count. SIRS describes the process of response by the body to an infection, such as with sepsis. It may eventually lead to septic shock and death if not managed appropriately.

Sepsis can develop following an infection and it can quickly lead to a life-threatening situation. A patient who is immunocompromised, such as someone who has cancer, is at higher risk of developing sepsis after an infection because his body is less likely to be able to fight off the infection. The patient described is at higher risk of other complications from his infection and from surgery because he has a history of leukemia, which puts him in a situation in which he is immunocompromised. The nurse would need to closely monitor this patient for signs of deterioration in clinical status that would indicate that he is becoming septic or developing shock.

Sepsis causes a number of changes in the body, which may be detected by lab results. When sepsis develops, the body reacts with an inflammatory response, causing vasodilation and increased capillary permeability. The person's blood pressure may drop because of the vasodilation and the nurse may see other changes, such as elevated glucose levels. This patient has leukemia, which would cause a change in blood cell levels as well, which is why he has altered levels of WBCs, RBCs, and platelets. In response to these lab results, the nurse should take measures to protect the patient's condition from worsening, monitor and try to restore his blood pressure, ensure that he has appropriate oxygenation, and keep him comfortable.

The patient who has developed sepsis is at risk of septic shock and death. Septic shock develops because of poor circulation and a drop in blood pressure. The patient may have such poor circulation and low blood pressure that he develops organ failure because the organs are not receiving enough blood. The patient in this example has a continued drop in blood pressure after surgery despite the administration of fresh frozen plasma. The physician would order a drug that would help to improve blood pressure to avoid septic shock and organ failure. The drug in this example is levophed, which is also a type of norepinephrine and is used as a vasoconstrictor to improve blood pressure.

The Swan-Ganz catheter is inserted as a central line and threaded to the interior of the heart to monitor internal blood pressure. Because this line is in place, the provider can continue to closely monitor the patient's hemodynamic status. The nurse must provide nearly constant care to this patient to prevent his further deterioration into shock and death. In this case, he has dropping blood pressure, which already indicates a clinical decline. Further measures must be taken to avoid organ failure, which can result from sepsis and septic shock.

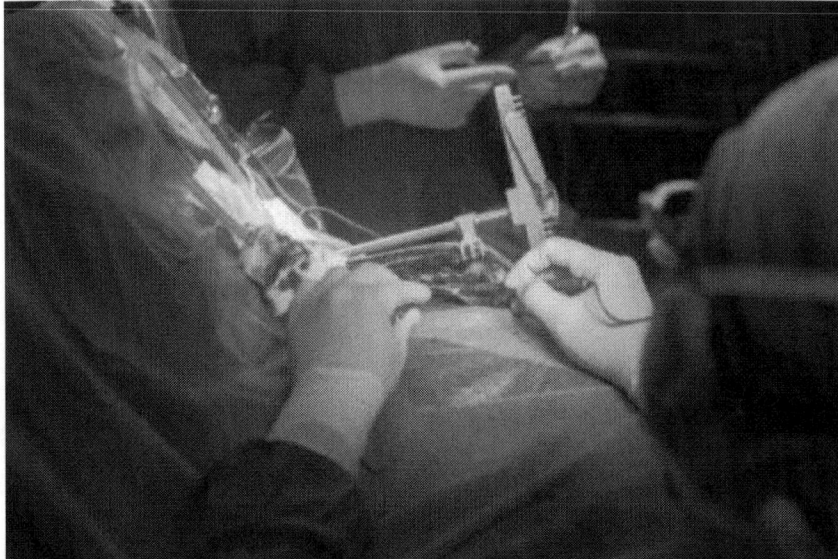

Ms. L is a 58-year-old female patient who is post-op day 1 after coronary artery bypass graft surgery (CABG). Ms. L has a history of coronary heart disease and angina; she recently had a coronary angiogram, which indicated that she had several blocked coronary arteries, ultimately necessitating the CABG. She spent the first day in the ICU after surgery and has just been transferred to the cardiac step-down unit where she is placed on telemetry. The nurse admitting Ms. L to the unit performs an assessment after receiving report; she notes the following vital signs: HR 108 bpm and irregular, RR 18/minute, BP 118/78 mmHg, O2 sat 98% on 1L O2 per nasal prongs. After connecting Ms. L to telemetry, the tech notes that she has an abnormal cardiac rhythm. Upon assessment of the cardiac monitor, the nurse notes that Ms. L is having periods of atrial fibrillation.

1. Discuss the potential for development of atrial fibrillation during the post-op period after CABG.

2. What measures would the nurse take that would prevent this patient from developing atrial fibrillation?

The nurse notifies the physician about Ms. L's condition and receives an order for 4mg warfarin. After giving the medication, the nurse continues to monitor the patient's cardiac rhythms with her assessments.

3.   What is the purpose of administering warfarin to a patient with atrial fibrillation?

4.   In addition to regular hemodynamic monitoring of the patient's cardiac status, what other tests or measures should the nurse monitor while the patient receives warfarin therapy?

Ms. L remains on the same amount of O2 per nasal cannula but has been unable to wean to a lesser amount. Each time the nursing staff try to decrease the amount of oxygen, the patient's saturations drop to between 86 and 89 percent. The nurse has given Ms. L a nursing diagnosis of Ineffective Airway Clearance related to her inability to wean from supplemental oxygen.

5. What are the most appropriate interventions the nurse would employ with this nursing diagnosis?

6. Describe atelectasis and its effects on respiratory patterns during the post-op period.

The nurse recognizes that Ms. L is having complications because she has avoided getting out of bed or participating in any activities. Each time the nurse tries to get Ms. L to sit up on the edge of the bed, she states that she is in too much pain to move.

7. Describe the potential complications that this particular patient is at risk for because of immobility.

8. How would the nurse intervene to increase the patient's mobility and so avoid some potential complications?

9. Provide three other examples of nursing diagnoses for Ms. L that are related to her condition.

Rationale

A person with severe heart disease that causes blockages in the coronary arteries may need surgery to prevent further arterial occlusion and an eventual heart attack. Coronary artery bypass graft (CABG) surgery is the process of rerouting blood flow around the blocked vessels in the heart so that the patient's heart muscle continues to receive oxygen and nutrients. During a CABG, a patient is usually placed on cardiopulmonary bypass, which continues to maintain circulatory function while the surgeon works on the heart. The surgeon removes a vessel from another part of the body, usually the leg, and sews in onto the heart to reroute blood flow around the blockage.

Following surgery, the patient is taken to the ICU, where she is closely monitored for cardiac function, respiratory patterns, and hemodynamic status. The nurse must remain alert for any signs of complications and intervene quickly before they become severe. This may mean checking for very subtle signs, such as small changes in vital signs or alterations in the patient's mental status. One potential complication following CABG surgery is development of cardiac dysrhythmias. Atrial fibrillation may occur in up to 50 percent of patients recovering from CABG surgery. During AF, the atria quiver and do not pump blood normally, putting the patient at risk of blood clots in the heart's chambers.

To prevent complications from AF, the nurse may administer anticoagulant medications, such as warfarin, to prevent blood clots, while administering other medications to control the heart rhythm. Warfarin increases the amount of time it takes the blood to clot, which can prevent blood clots from forming but can also increase the patient's risk of bleeding. When giving warfarin, the nurse must monitor for signs of bleeding, such as easy bruising or petechiae or oozing from the incision site. Regular warfarin administration also includes routine laboratory testing for clotting times, such as by checking PT, PTT, or INR levels.

Because CABG surgery is so significant, the patient will have an extensive recovery in front of her. However, it is still important to provide range-of-motion exercises and maintain some levels of activity to prevent complications of immobility. A patient recovering from cardiac surgery may want to stay in bed but it is important to get up and move to avoid the risk of blood clots, skin breakdown, and lung atelectasis that can happen with immobility. In this case, if the patient has not been getting up much and has not been using spirometry, she is at high risk of atelectasis following surgery, which occurs as some of the alveoli of the lungs collapse and deflate. The patient will suffer poor oxygenation because she has fewer alveoli to promote gas exchange.

The nurse must work to prevent complications after cardiac surgery, including those affecting the cardiovascular system and those related to immobility. This involves very detailed management of the patient's condition, such as by administering pain medications, helping the client to get up and ambulate, monitoring breathing rate and hemodynamic status, and ensuring the patient receives adequate nutrition. This patient requires high levels of nursing care during the post-op period and would have several nursing diagnoses in place. Some examples of appropriate nursing diagnoses in this situation would include Activity Intolerance, Alteration in Comfort, Alteration in Nutrition: Less than Body Requirements, Knowledge Deficit, and Altered Tissue Perfusion, among others.

Pancreatitis

A 44-year-old male patient has been admitted to the medical-surgical unit of the hospital for after seeking treatment for nausea, vomiting, and severe abdominal pain. The patient developed sudden and intense pain in the right upper quadrant the evening before and waited for a few hours before seeking treatment. He has a history of substance abuse and has been in rehabilitation for both alcohol and stimulant abuse. He currently still uses both alcohol and methamphetamines, despite previous attempts of treatment at detoxification centers.

Upon admission, the patient is anxious and restless, complaining of severe pain that is unrelieved by pain medication. The nurse contacts the physician to ask for further orders for opioid medications to treat the pain. The physician also orders further diagnostic tests to confirm the cause of the patient's pain and symptoms, as well as a 500 mL bolus of lactated Ringer's solution IV, followed by a regular rate of LR at 150 mL/hour.

1. What types of diagnostic tests would most likely be ordered that could determine the cause of this type of abdominal pain?

2. What laboratory tests would the physician most likely order?

3. What effects would the patient's history of drug and alcohol abuse have on his abdominal pain?

The physician orders an abdominal ultrasound and several laboratory tests, including a CBC, metabolic panel, glucose, serum amylase, and serum lipase. The nurse is also given an order for IV fentanyl to be given prn every 4 hours for pain control. After undergoing the ultrasound, the physician considers that the patient may have acute pancreatitis caused by inflammation; there are several lesions noted on the pancreas that may have been caused by chronic alcohol use.

4. Based on the diagnosis of acute pancreatitis, what changes in laboratory values would the nurse expect to see in this patient?

5. Why is pain control such an important component of management of acute pancreatitis?

Following diagnosis and continued administration of pain medications, the patient is still complaining of pain. The nurse notes several areas of petechiae on his abdomen, particularly in the right upper quadrant. While once complaining vocally about the pain, the patient now is more quiet, lethargic, grimacing, and guarding the abdomen. His vital signs are: HR: 102 bpm, RR: 22/min, BP: 94/68 mmHg, T: 101.0°F. The nurse contacts the physician, who leaves orders for blood pressure support medications, supplemental oxygen, and antibiotics. The patient is transferred to the ICU for further care.

6. In addition to contacting the physician, how should the nurse intervene in this situation?

7. What types of complications do the patient's signs and symptoms indicate?

Rationale

Pancreatitis describes inflammation that occurs in the pancreas; it can develop as a short-term condition, which is treated and resolved and is classified as acute, or as a long-term condition known as chronic pancreatitis. The most common cause of both acute and chronic pancreatitis is alcohol abuse. Among those who develop acute pancreatitis, alcohol abuse is the second most common cause of the condition. It is thought that continued abuse of alcohol can increase the risk of the pancreas becoming injured or infected when combined with other factors; alcohol abuse is also thought to cause lesions on the surface of the pancreas that can contribute to inflammation and disease.

The pancreas is important for secreting digestive enzymes that break down certain types of foods and for creating and secreting insulin in response to blood glucose levels. When a person presents for care with symptoms that can indicate pancreatitis, he will most likely be suffering from acute pain in the right upper quadrant of the abdomen. Nausea, vomiting, fever, and tachycardia are other signs and symptoms that are also present with acute pancreatitis. Although the patient in this situation most likely developed pancreatitis because of alcohol abuse, there are other factors that can contribute to the condition. Gallstones are the most common cause of acute pancreatitis, but the condition can also develop because of injury to the pancreas, chronically high cholesterol levels, high blood calcium levels, or because of drug use or infection.

Diagnosis of pancreatitis often includes imaging tests, such as an ultrasound or abdominal CT to identify the inflammation. Laboratory testing usually checks for the presence of infection in the body by testing the level of white blood cells; the physician may also order levels of pancreatic enzymes, including amylase and lipase; a calcium level, since hypercalcemia can cause pancreatitis, and a glucose level may be needed since the pancreas is responsible for secreting insulin.

Treatment of pancreatitis typically involves administration of IV fluids, and may require a bolus of fluid to prevent dehydration and to reduce high concentrations of certain types of electrolytes in the bloodstream. Because the patient usually experiences pain, the nurse would also need to provide pain medication, often in the form of opioid medications given IV. A patient who has pain that is not well treated is at risk for other complications of pancreatitis and may have a harder time fully healing from the condition.

A small percentage of patients with acute pancreatitis may develop severe acute pancreatitis (SAP) which can be life threatening and can lead to shock, organ failure, and death. The nurse should be aware of the potential for SAP and should monitor for signs and symptoms that indicate that the patient is going into shock, such as a drop in blood pressure, decreased urine output, and abnormal bleeding. Rapid management of SAP is important by providing fluid resuscitation, antibiotics, nutrition, pain control, and blood pressure control to prevent the patient from deteriorating and to improve his chances of survival.

Respiratory Acidosis

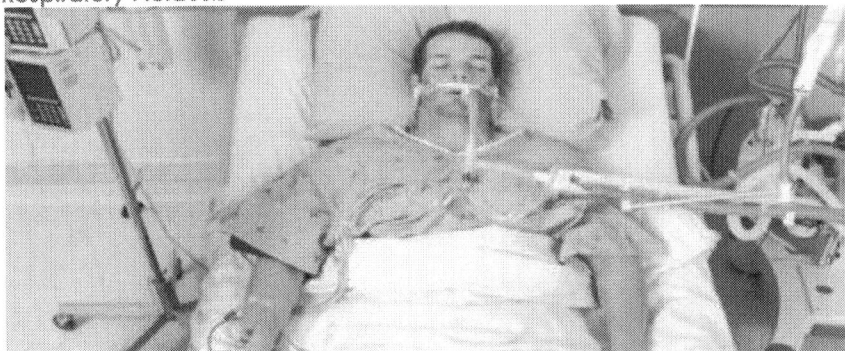

E. P. is a 21-year-old female patient who was brought in to the hospital after suffering minor burns from a fire in the college dorm where she lives. E. P. has several superficial burns noted on her right forearm; she says she bumped against a burning door while trying to leave the building. She does not have a history of any medical conditions or illnesses, except surgery for an appendectomy when she was 10 years old. She arrives at the hospital accompanied by a friend from her school.

During the assessment, E. P. is anxious and is breathing rapidly, her skin is warm and flushed and she appears anxious. Her HR is 110 bpm and she is breathing at a rate of 32/minute but is taking shallow breaths. Her BP is 98/68 mmHg and her oxygen saturations are 94% on room air. The nurse starts an IV as ordered by the physician and administers pain medication for the burns. She places E. P. on oxygen by nasal cannula at a rate of 2 L/minute to keep oxygen saturations over 95%.

1. The patient's respiratory rate is rapid and shallow. Over time, how will this breathing pattern affect the patient's circulation?

2. What types of laboratory tests might the physician order for this patient?

The nurse dresses the patient's wounds on her arm but notes that E. P. continues to breathe in a rapid and shallow manner. Despite 2L of oxygen, her saturations remain low. E. P. now appears confused and can't seem to remember now why she is in the hospital. The physician believes she may have experienced smoke inhalation because of the fire. He orders a chest x-ray, ABG, metabolic panel, and lactic acid level and the nurse sets up to assist with rapid sequence intubation. The results of the ABG are as follows: pH 7.31, pCO_2 49 mmHg, pO_2 80 mmHg, HCO_3 24 mmHg. The lactic acid level is 8.6 mmol/L.

3. What do these ABG results indicate?

4. Why is the lactic acid level elevated?

5. Why would the physician choose to perform rapid sequence intubation in this case?

6. How would the nurse assist the physician during rapid sequence intubation?

The patient is intubated and placed on mechanical ventilation, using FiO2 of 60%. The staff prepare to send her to the ICU for ongoing care. The nurse has given E.P. a nursing diagnosis of Ineffective Airway Clearance related to smoke inhalation as evidenced by altered respiratory patterns, decreased oxygen saturations, and respiratory acidosis demonstrated on the ABG.

7.   Which nursing interventions would the nurse employ for a diagnosis of Ineffective Airway Clearance?

Rationale

Respiratory acidosis is an altered state characterized by an acid-base imbalance in the bloodstream; it develops when a person's carbon dioxide levels in the blood are elevated and the pH of the blood is low. Acute respiratory acidosis can develop for a number of reasons, including hypoxia due to conditions such as smoke inhalation, as well as other situations, such as pneumonia, drug overdose, pulmonary edema, or chest wall trauma. Untreated, the patient with severe respiratory acidosis could eventually develop shock and go into cardiac arrest.

This patient's breathing patterns are abnormal; she is breathing too fast and at a shallow rate, which means that she is probably retaining too much carbon dioxide in the bloodstream. This is evidenced by the ABG results, which show a high level of CO_2 but also a normal level of bicarbonate, meaning that she is suffering from a respiratory condition and not a metabolic condition. The pH is low, which indicates acidosis. The lactic acid level is elevated, which better confirms smoke inhalation in this patient, based on her ABG results and medical history. Elevated lactic acid levels in the bloodstream mean that body tissues are not getting enough oxygen.

Rapid sequence intubation (RSI) describes the process of inserting an endotracheal tube while simultaneously administering sedative agents. RSI is performed when intubation is emergent and the patient needs respiratory support right away. In this case, the patient's health is deteriorating, as evidenced by respiratory acidosis as seen on the ABG results, her inability to maintain normal oxygen saturations despite administration of supplemental oxygen, and her changes in cognitive status. Waiting to intubate this patient could also increase the risk of difficulties with intubation later; since the patient suffered from smoke inhalation, she could experience swelling in the trachea, which would make it difficult to pass an ET tube.

Normally, the physician or anesthesia provider who is leading the RSI would administer many of the medications, because they often include neuromuscular blocking agents that would be used during anesthesia of surgery, although the nurse may administer some medications that are indicated, such as opioid analgesics or muscle relaxant medications. Additionally, the provider will most likely be the person who will pass the ET tube. The nurse's role is to ensure that all equipment the provider will need is ready and at hand when he needs it. She should be available with suction in case the patient has excess secretions, she should provide cricoid pressure if indicated, and she should watch the monitor to keep a close eye on the patient's hemodynamic status during the process. Following intubation, the nurse may provide breaths with a bag-valve device and work with a respiratory therapist to set up the ventilator and manage its settings.

A nurse who is caring for a patient with a nursing diagnosis of Ineffective Airway Clearance would have a number of nursing interventions in order to best monitor the patient's condition and prevent it from worsening. The nurse should routinely monitor the patient's respiratory effort by checking the rate and character of respirations as well as auscultating lung sounds, she would need to manage the ventilator and provide endotracheal suction when needed. The nurse would also need to monitor other clinical signs of deterioration that would be affected by poor gas exchange, such as signs of poor circulation, changes in mental status, cool and pale extremities, poor peripheral pulses, or an elevated or decreased heart rate. If any of these signs or symptoms occur, the nurse must be familiar with appropriate interventions to respond rapidly and prevent further deterioration. The nurse may need to administer some medications that would improve the patient's ability to breathe, such as bronchodilator medications. Additionally, part of ongoing care of the patient on a ventilator would be to continue to monitor oxygenation, including through oxygen saturations, and increase or decrease the FiO_2 as needed.

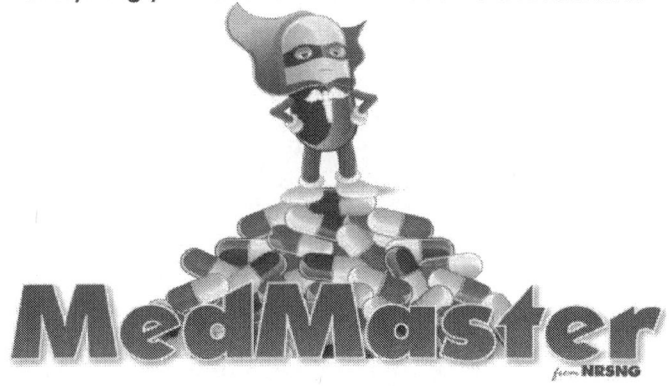

36 Nursing Cheat Sheets
for Students
NRSNG.com | NursingStudentBooks.com
Jon Haws RN CCRN
Sandra Haws RD CNSC
© TazKai LLC 2015

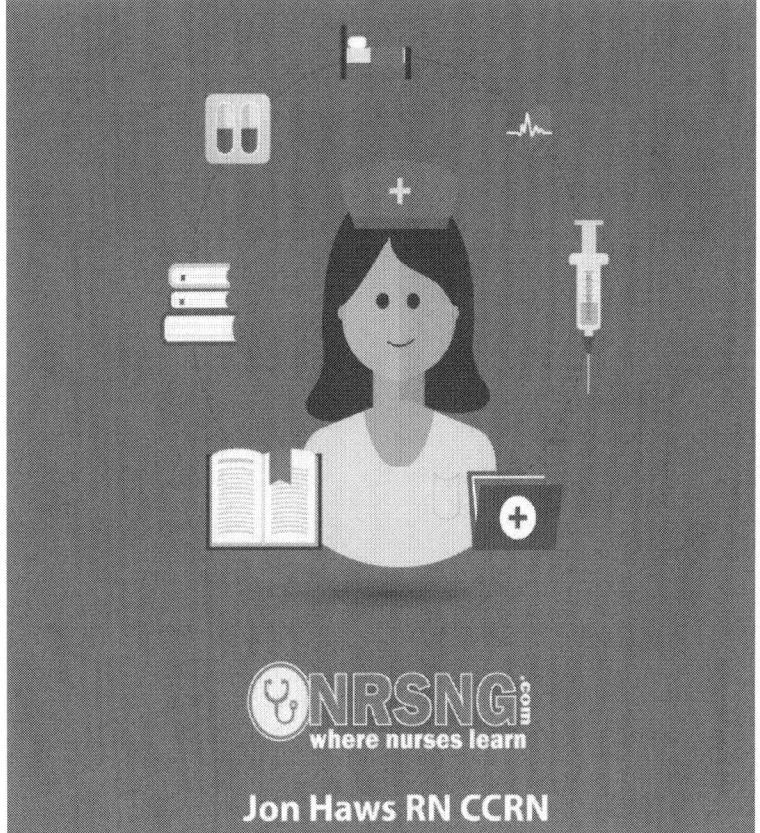

36 NURSING

Cheat Sheets for Students

NRSNG.com
where nurses learn

Jon Haws RN CCRN

Introduction

First of all . . . THANKS! Thank you for supporting NRSNG.com and for sharing our mission of improving nursing education. My journey into nursing was a long one but I have found it to be a truly rewarding career that allows me to make a difference and have ample family time. I am confident that you will achieve your goals. The fact that you are seeking additional resources to improve your understanding speaks volumes to your dedication. Second of all, this book is intended to provide you with a quick reference to some of the most needed and most used information for nursing students.

This is not a complete guide to nursing but a simple and compact quick reference to some of the most important information.

As always you should consult institutional policies when it comes to patient care.

Happy Nursing!

-Jon Haws RN CCRN
NRSNG.com | NursingStudentBooks.com

Injection Sites (IM)

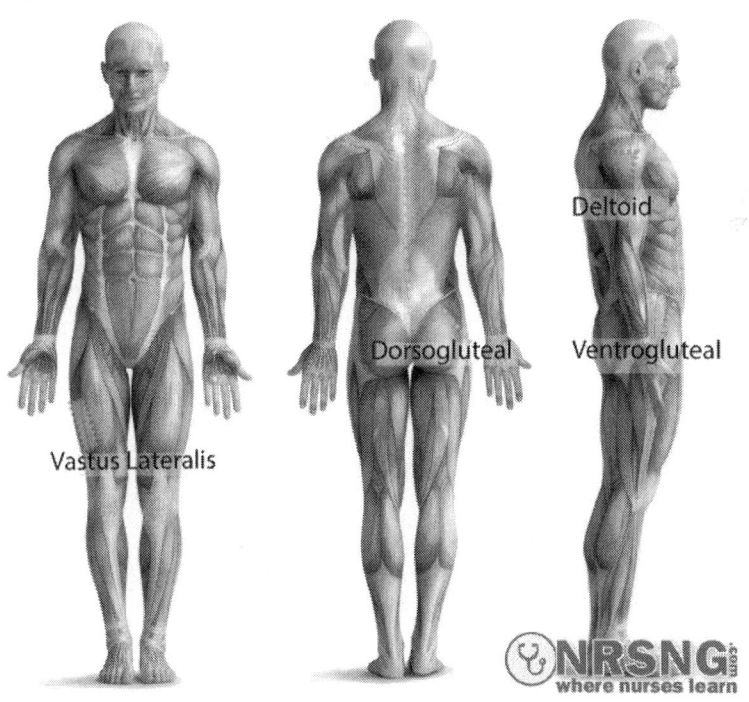

Deltoid

Dorsogluteal

Ventrogluteal

Vastus Lateralis

Common Laboratory Values

Complete Blood Count (CBC) with Differential

Value	Abbreviation	Unit	Normal Range
Red Blood Cell	RBC	x10^6/ml	Male: 4.5 - 5.5 Female: 4.0 - 4.9
White Blood Cell	WBC	cells/mcL	4,500 - 10,000
Neutrophils			54 - 62%
Band Forms			3 - 5% (>8% = left shift)
Eosinophils			1 - 3%
Basophils			0 - 0.75%
Lymphocytes			25 - 33%
Monocytes			3 - 7%
Platelets	PLT	cells/mcL	100,000 - 450,000
Hemoglobin	Hgb	g/dl	Male: 13.5 - 16.5 Female: 12.0 - 15.0
Hematocrit	Hct	%	Male: 41 - 50 Female: 36 - 44
Mean Corpuscular Volume	MCV	fL	80 - 100
Red Cell Distribution Width	RDW		<14.5

Blood Chemistry (Basic Metabolic Panel) (BMP)

Value	Abbreviation	Unit	Normal Range
Sodium	Na+	mEq/L	135 - 145
Potassium	K+	mEq/L	3.5 - 5.5
Chloride	Cl-	mEq/L	96 - 108
Glucose	Glu	mg/dL	70 - 115
Calcium	Ca^2+	mg/dL	8.4 - 10.2
Creatinine	Cr	mg/L	0.7 - 1.40
Blood Urea Nitrogen	BUN	mg/dL	7-20

Coagulation Studies

Value	Abbreviation	Unit	Normal
Prothrombin Time	PT	Seconds	11 - 14
Partial Thromboplastin Time	PTT	Seconds	25 - 35
International Normalized Ratio	INR		0.8 - 1.2
Activated Partial Thromboplastin Time	aPTT		1.5 - 2.5

Cholesterol Levels

Value	Abbreviation	Unit	Normal
Cholesterol Total		mg/dL	<200
Low Density Lipoprotein	LDL	mg/dL	<70
High Density Lipoprotein	HDL	mg/dL	<60 optimal
Triglycerides		mg/dL	<150

Arterial Blood Gas

Value	Abbreviation	Unit	Normal
pH	pH		7.35 - 7.45
Partial Pressure of CO_2	pCO_2	mmHg	35 - 45
Partial Pressure of O_2	pO_2	mmHg	80 - 100
Bicarbonate	HCO_3	mEq/L	22 - 26
Base Excess	BE	mEq/L	-2 - +2
Oxygen Saturation	SaO_2	%	95 - 100

Blood Gas Analysis

Value	Normal Range	What does it mean?
pH	7.34-7.44	The pH or H+ indicates if a patient is acidemic (pH < 7.35; H+ >45) or alkalemic (pH > 7.45; H+ < 35).
Arterial oxygen partial pressure (PaO2)	75-100 mmHg	A low PaO2 indicates that the patient is not oxygenating properly, and is hypoxemic. (Note that a low PaO2 is not required for the patient to have hypoxia.) At a PaO2 of less than 60 mm Hg, supplemental oxygen should be administered. At a PaO2 of less than 26 mmHg, the patient is at risk of death and must be oxygenated immediately
Arterial carbon dioxide partial pressure (PaCO2)	35-45 mmHg	The carbon dioxide partial pressure (PaCO2) is an indicator of CO2 production and elimination: for a constant metabolic rate, the PaCO2 is determined entirely by its elimination through ventilation.[9] A high PaCO2 (respiratory acidosis, alternatively hypercapnia) indicates underventilation (or, more rarely, a hypermetabolic disorder), a low PaCO2 (respiratory alkalosis, alternatively hypocapnia) hyper- or overventilation.
HCO3-	22-26 mEq/L	The HCO3- ion indicates whether a metabolic problem is present (such as ketoacidosis). A low HCO3- indicates metabolic acidosis, a high HCO3- indicates metabolic alkalosis. As this value when given with blood gas results is often calculated by the analyzer, correlation should be checked with total CO2 levels as directly measured.
Base excess	-2 to +2 mmol/L	The base excess is used for the assessment of the metabolic component of acid-base disorders, and indicates whether the patient has metabolic acidosis or metabolic alkalosis. Contrasted with the bicarbonate levels, the base excess is a calculated value intended to completely isolate the non-respiratory portion of the pH change. There are two calculations for base excess (extra cellular fluid - BE(ecf); blood - BE(b)). The calculation used for the BE(ecf) = cHCO3 - 24.8 +16.2 X (pH-7.4). The calculation used for BE(b) = (1-0.014 x hgb) x (cHCO3 - 24.8 + (1.43 x hgb + 7.7) x (pH -7.4).

Blood Gas Interpretation

Respiratory Acidosis	pH	$PaCO_2$	HCO_3
Acute	< 7.35	> 45	Normal
Partly Compensated	< 7.35	> 45	> 26
Compensated	Normal	> 45	> 26
Respiratory Alkalosis			
Acute	> 7.45	< 35	Normal
Partly Compensated	> 7.45	< 35	< 22
Compensated	Normal	< 35	< 22
Metabolic Acidosis			
Acute	< 7.35	Normal	< 22
Partly Compensated	< 7.35	< 35	< 22
Compensated	Normal	< 35	< 22
Metabolic Alkalosis			
Acute	> 7.45	Normal	> 26
Partly Compensated	> 7.45	> 45	> 26
Compensated	Normal	> 45	> 26

Blood Compatibility

Blood Group	Antigens	Antibodies	Can give blood (RBC) to	Can receive blood (RBC) from
AB	A and B	None	AB	AB, A, B, O
A	A	B	A and AB	A and O
B	B	A	B and AB	B and O
O	None	A and B	AB, A, B, O	O

Anticoagulant Therapy

Lab values for individuals on anticoagulant therapy
INR: 2-3 dependant on indication
(http://www.globalrph.com/warfarin_inr_targets.htm)

$$INR = \frac{PT_{test}}{PT_{normal}}$$

Heart Murmurs

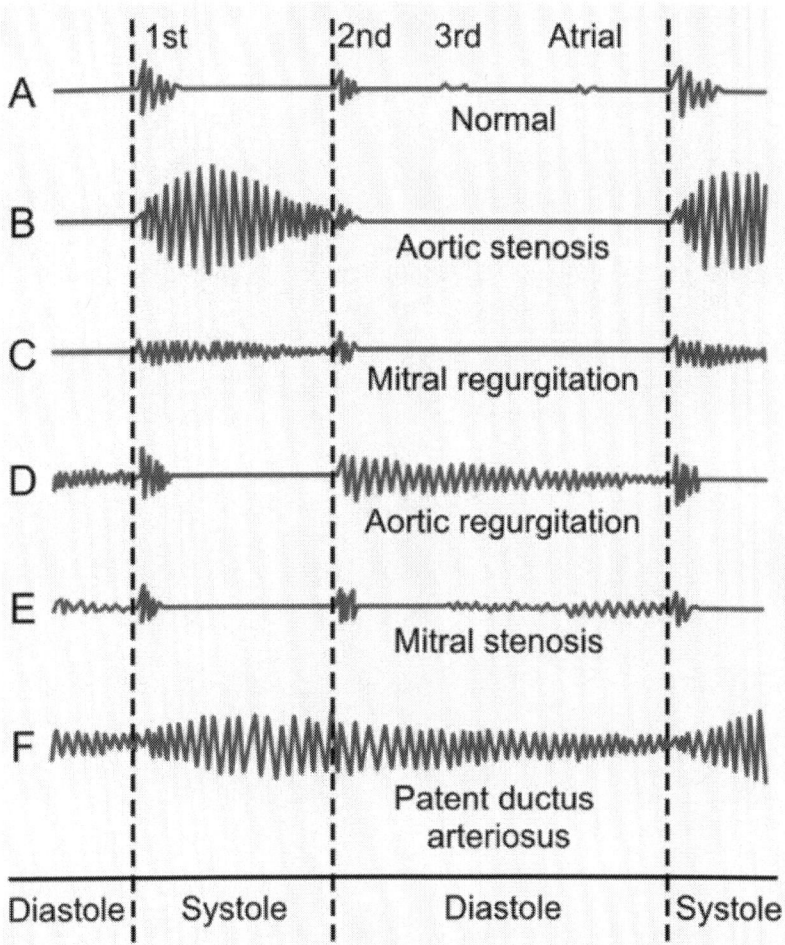

Phonocardiograms from normal and abnormal heart sounds

Glasgow Coma Scale

	1	2	3	4	5	6
Eye	Does not open	Opens to painful stimuli	Opens to voice	Opens spontaneously	N/A	N/A
Verbal	Makes no sound	Incomprehensible sounds	Utters inappropriate words	Confused, disoriented	Oriented	N/A
Motor	No movement	Extension to painful stimuli (decerebrate response)	Abnormal flexion to painful stimuli (decorticate response)	Withdraws to painful stimuli	Localizes to painful stimuli	Obeys commands

Cranial Nerves

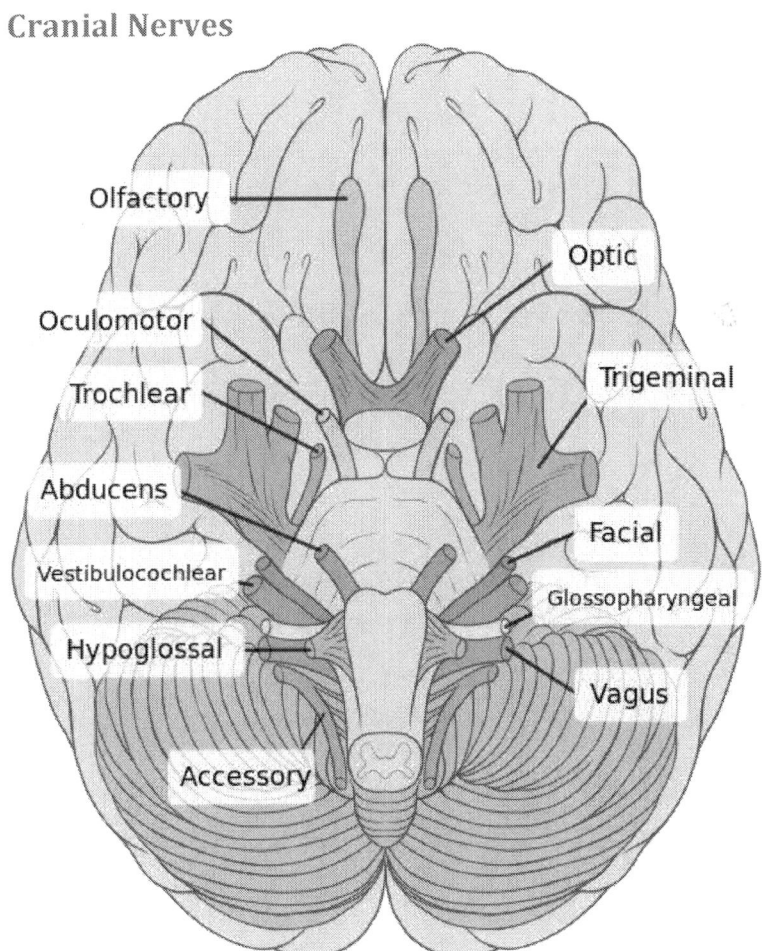

Wallace Rule of Nines - Burn Severity

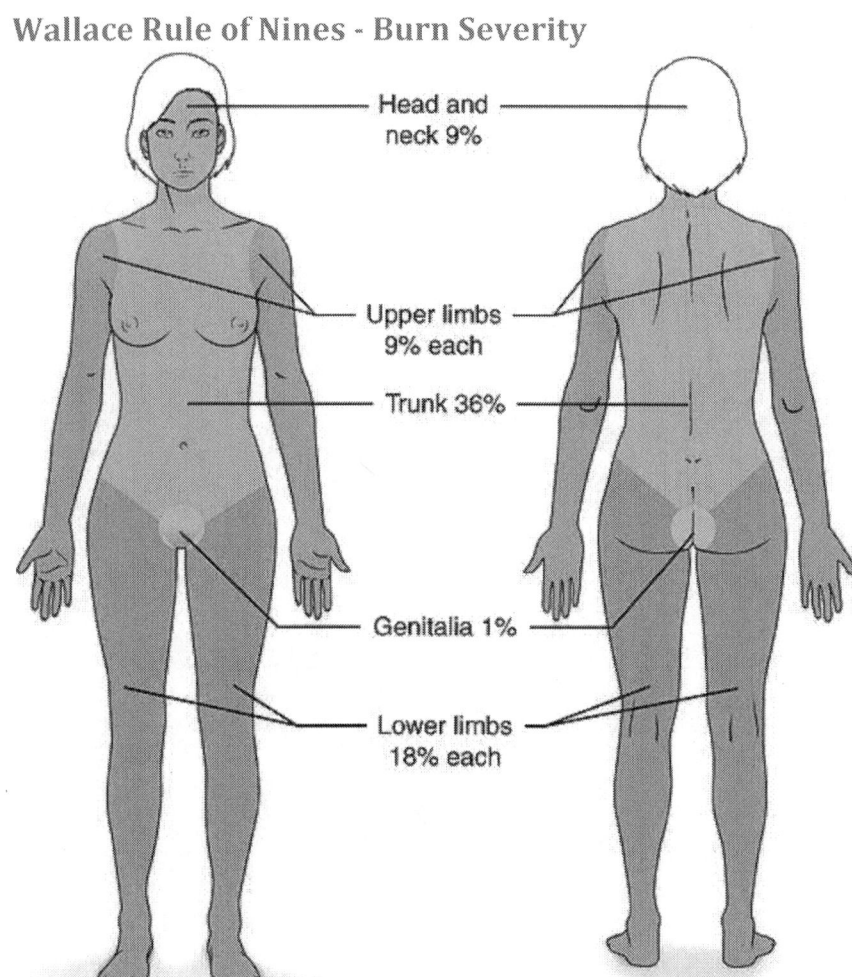

Edema Scale

1+: Mild: both feet/ankles
2+: Moderate: both feet, plus lower legs, hands or lower arms
3+: Severe: generalized bilateral pitting edema, including both feet, legs, arms, and face
4+: >30 seconds to rebound

Wigger Diagram

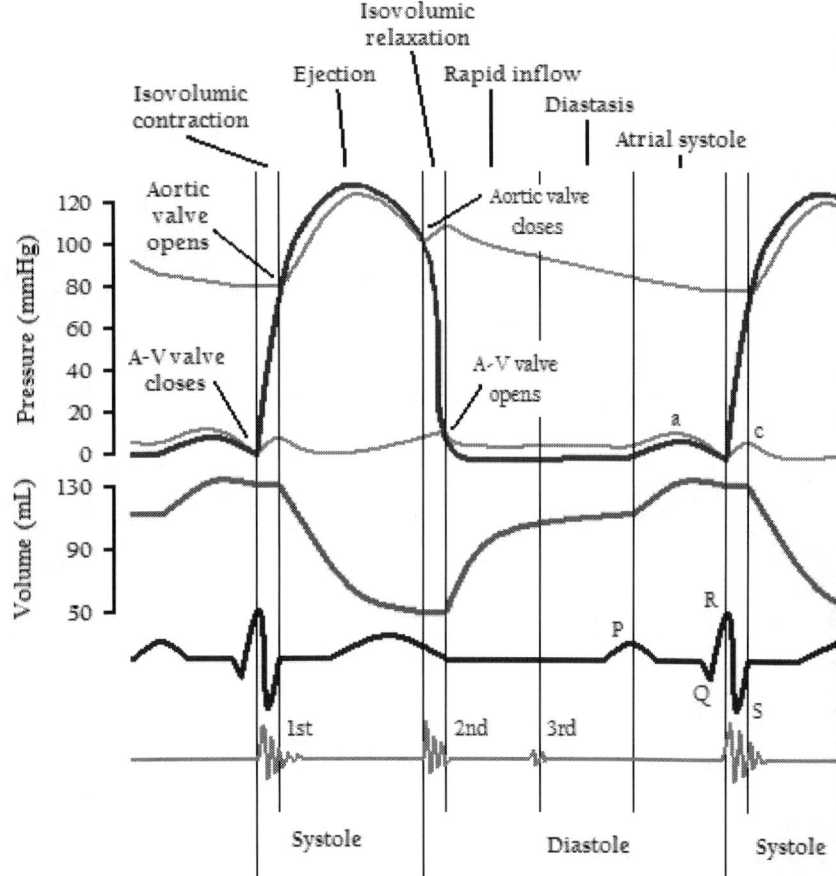

Correspondence between valves, beats, pressures, and sounds within the heart.

Heart Sounds

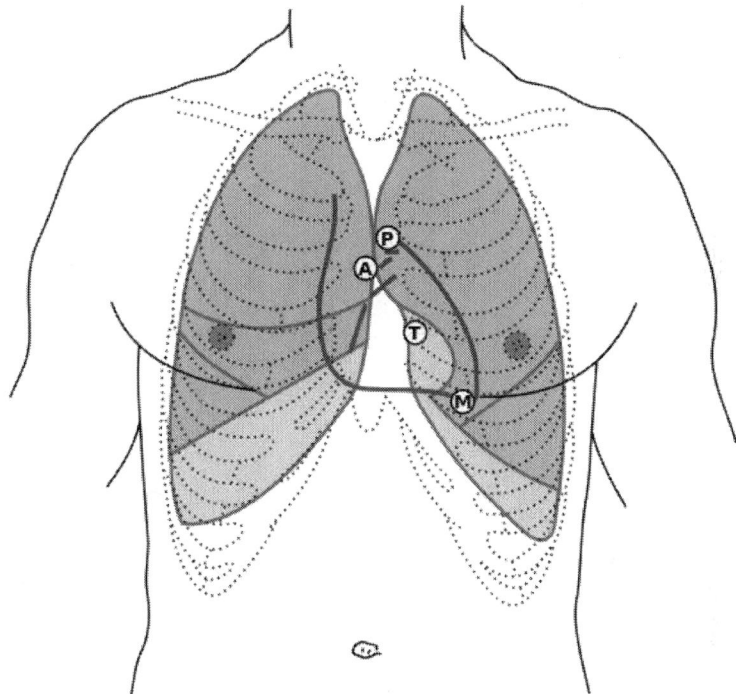

Locations for listening to heart sounds: **APE To Man**

Normal EKG

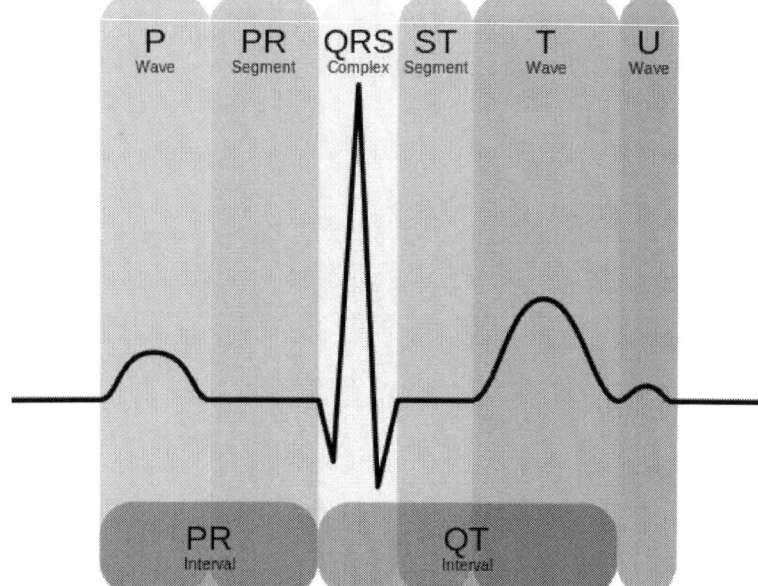

12 Lead EKG Placement

EKG Strip Interpretation

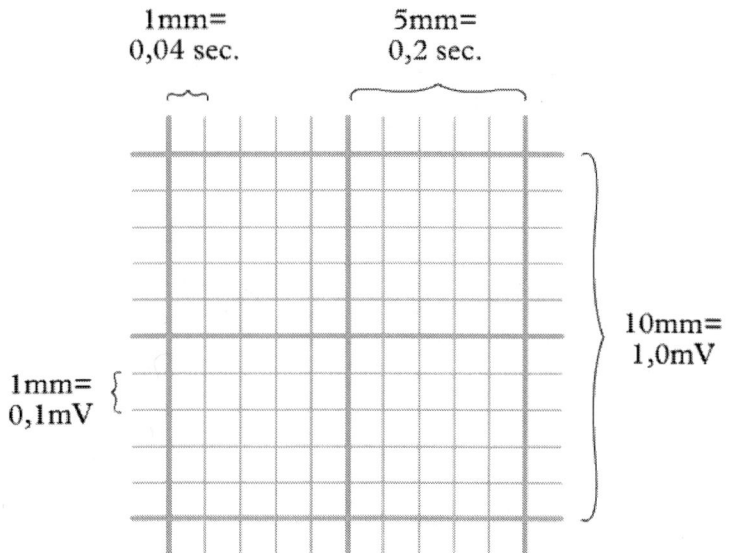

1mm=
0,04 sec.

5mm=
0,2 sec.

10mm=
1,0mV

1mm=
0,1mV

Abnormal EKG
STEMI V1 - V5 notice the ST elevation in leads V1 - V5

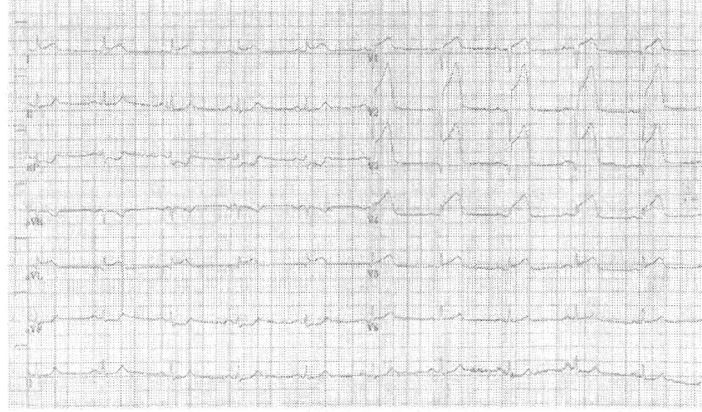

Ventricular Tachycardia

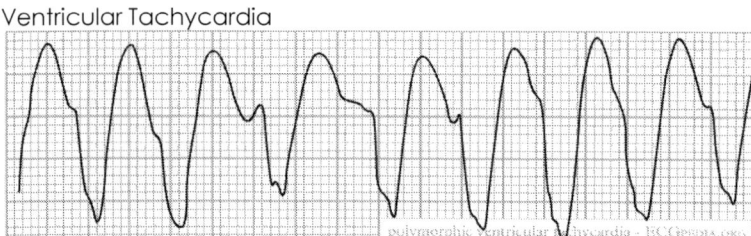

polymorphic ventricular tachycardia - ECGpedia.org

PCV - notice the early ventricular beat

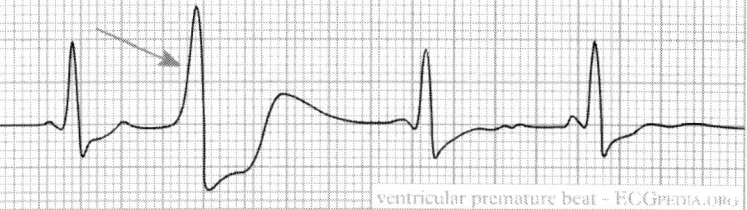

ventricular premature beat - ECGPEDIA.ORG

Atrial Flutter

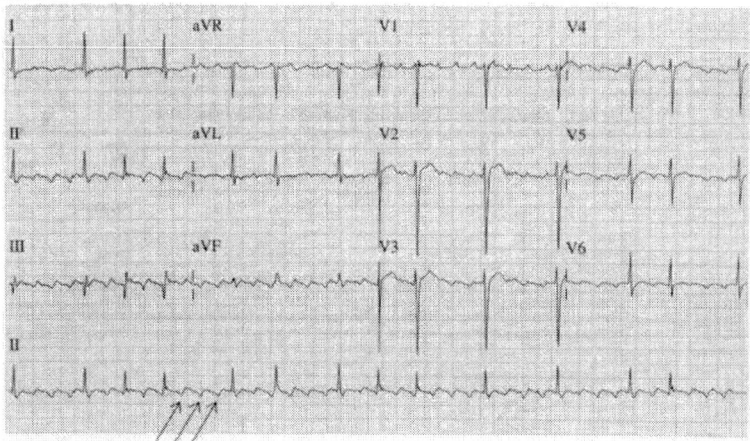

Atrial Fibrillation with RVR

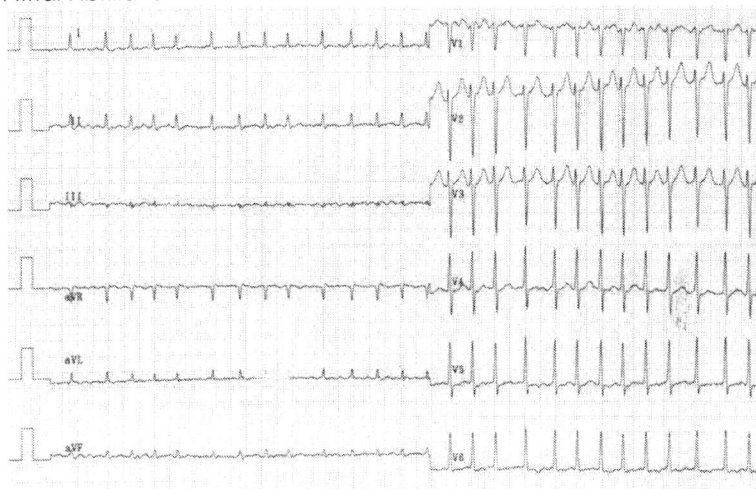

5 Lead EKG Placement

White on Right (arm) - Black on Left (arm)
Green on Right (ABD or leg) - Red on Left (ABD or leg)

Mnemonic:
Snow over Trees - Smoke over Fire

Heart Murmurs

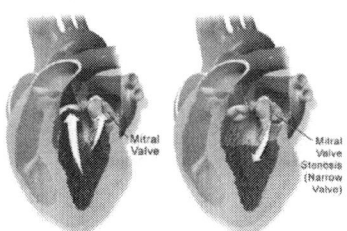

Mitral Valve Regurgitation   Mitral Valve Stenosis

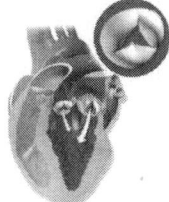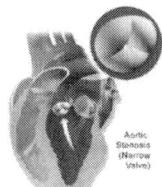

Aortic Regurgitation   Aortic Stenosis

	AORTIC	MITRAL
SYSTOLE	OPEN STENOSIS	CLOSED REGURGITATION
DIASTOLE	CLOSED REGURGITATION	OPEN STENOSIS

Shock

The goal of the cardio-pulmonary system is to deliver O2 to the body

Shock is a state of vital organs not receiving adequate O2

3 Main Types of Shock

> Hypovolemic - Low volume
> Cardiogenic - Broken pump (heart)
> Septic - Immune response interferes with vascular tone

Normal Oxygen Delivery System

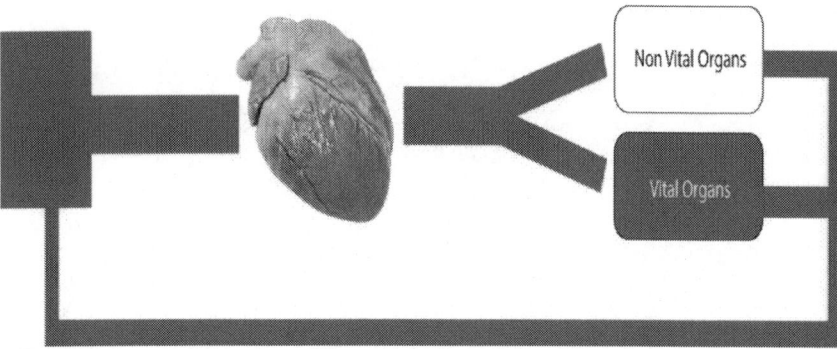

With each type of shock a different portion of the O2 deliver system is effected:

Hypovolemic - The initial insult is low blood volume

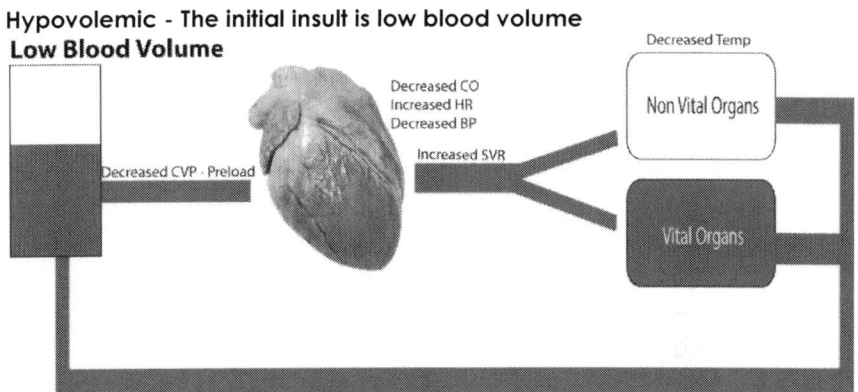

Low Blood Volume

Decreased CO
Increased HR
Decreased BP

Increased SVR

Decreased CVP - Preload

Decreased Temp

Non Vital Organs

Vital Organs

Hypovolemic Shock Stages:

Class I: 500-750 ml loss
Class II: 750-1500 ml loss
Class III: 1500-2000 ml loss
Class IV: >2000 ml

Cardiogenic - Initial insult is pump failure

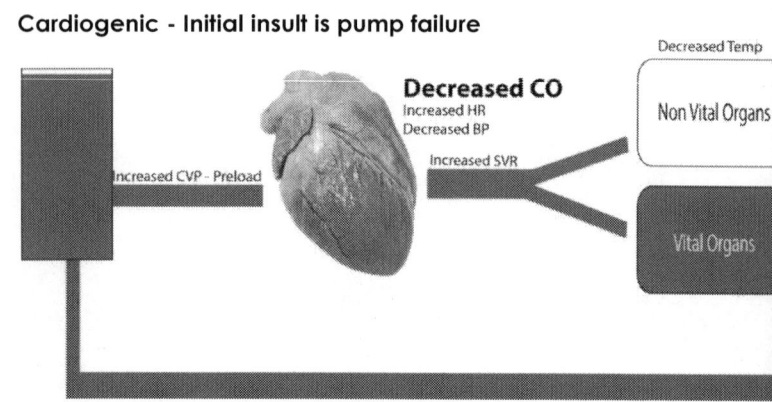

Decreased Temp

Decreased CO
Increased HR
Decreased BP

Non Vital Organs

Increased CVP - Preload

Increased SVR

Vital Organs

Septic - Immune response (inflammation) initiates systemic vasodilation

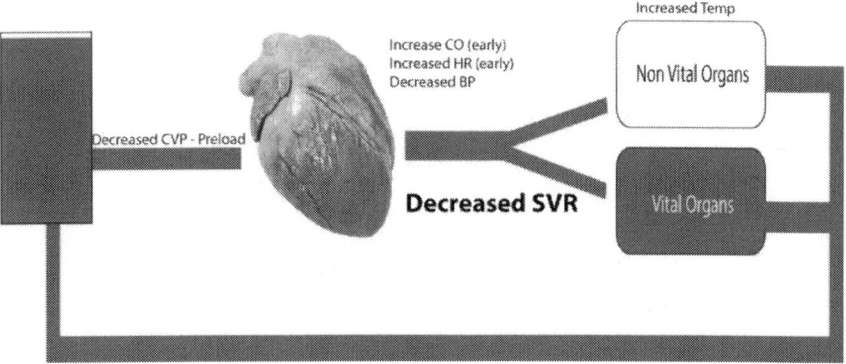

Increased Temp

Increase CO (early)
Increased HR (early)
Decreased BP

Non Vital Organs

Decreased CVP - Preload

Decreased SVR

Vital Organs

Comparison of Different Types of Shock (NOT all inclusive)

	Hypovolemic	Cardiogenic	Septic
CO	↓	↓ Initial Insult	↑ (early)
HR	↑	↑	↑ (early)
SVR	↑	↑	↓ Initial Insult
EF	↑	↓	↓
PAOP (L Atria)	↓	↑	↓
CVP R Preload	↓ Initial Insult	↑	↓
BP	↓	↓	↓
Temp	↓	↓	↑

Hierarchy of O2 Delivery

Nasal Cannula
1 lpm = 24%
2 lpm = 28%
3 lpm = 32%
4 lpm = 36%
5 lpm = 40%
6 lpm = 44%
Simple Face Mask
5 lpm = 40%
6 lpm = 45-50%
7 lpm = 50-55%
8 lpm = 55-60%
Non-rebreather Mask
6 lpm = 60%
7 lpm = 70%
8 lpm = 80%
9 lpm = 90%
10 lpm = close to 100%
Venturi Mask
4 lpm = 24-28%
8 lpm = 35-40%
12 lpm = 50%
Trach Collar
21-70% at 10L
T-Piece
21-100% with flow rate at 2.5 times minute ventilation
CPAP
Positive airway pressure during spontaneous breaths
Bi-PAP
Positive pressure during spontaneous breaths and preset pressure to be maintained during expiration
SIMV
Preset Vt and f. Circuit remains open between mandatory breaths so pt can take additional breaths. Ventilator doesn't cycle during spontaneous breaths so Vt varies. Mandatory breaths synchronized so they do not occur during spontaneous breaths.
Assist Control
Preset Vt and f and inspiratory effort required to assist spontaneous breaths. Delivers control breaths. Cycles additionally if pt inspiratory effort is adequate. Same Vt delivered for spontaneous breaths.

(http://web.missouri.edu/~danneckere/pt316/case/pulm/FiO2.htm)

(http://web.missouri.edu/~danneckere/pt316/case/pulm/FiO2.htm)

http://www.ucdenver.edu/academics/colleges/medicalschool/departments/medicine/intmed/imrp/CURRICULUM/Documents/Oxygenation%20and%20oxygen%20therapy.pdf

Wound (Pressure Ulcer) Staging

I

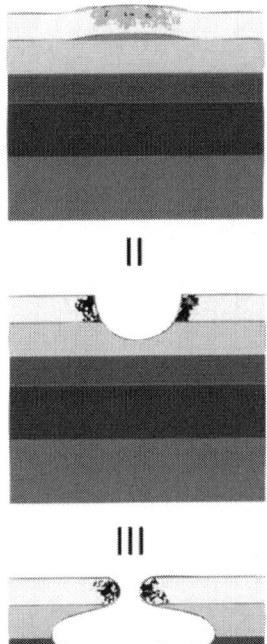

II

III

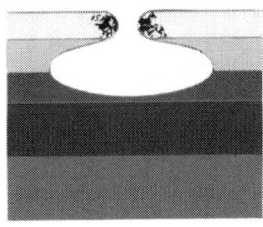

IV

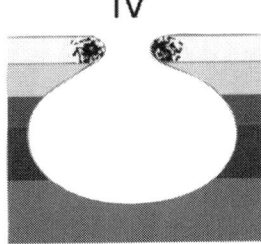

IV Fluid Therapy

One liter of Ringers Lactate solution contains:
130 mEq of sodium ion = 130 mmol/L
109 mEq of chloride ion = 109 mmol/L
28 mEq of lactate = 28 mmol/L
4 mEq of potassium ion = 4 mmol/L
3 mEq of calcium ion = 1.5 mmol/L

One liter of 0.9% Saline contains:
154 mEq of sodium ion = 154 mmol/L
154 mEq of chloride ion = 154 mmol/L

One liter "banana bag" contains 1L of normal saline (sodium chloride 0.9%) with:

Thiamine 100 mg
Folic acid 1 mg
MVI 1 amp (Multivitamin for infusion, 1 ampule)
3 grams of magnesium sulfate

Medication Antidotes

Medication	Antidote
Tylenol	Acetylcysteine (mucomyst)
Potassium	Insulin, $NaHCO_3$, Kayexalate, albuterol
Iron	Deferoxamine
Digoxin	Digiband
Benzodiazepines	Flumazenil (Romazicon)
Magnesium Sulfate	Calcium Gluconate
Opioids	Naloxone (Narcan)
Narcotics	Naloxone (Narcan)
Heparin	Protamine Sulfate
Coumadin	Vitamin K

Insulin Onset, Peak, and Durations

Type of Insulin	Brand Name	Generic Name	Onset	Peak	Duration
Rapid-acting	NovoLog	Insulin aspart	15 minutes	30 to 90 minutes	3 to 5 hours
	Apidra	Insulin glulisine	15 minutes	30 to 90 minutes	3 to 5 hours
	Humalog	Insulin lispro	15 minutes	30 to 90 minutes	3 to 5 hours
Short-acting	Humulin R Novolin R	Regular (R)	30 to 60 minutes	2 to 4 hours	5 to 8 hours
Intermediate-acting	Humulin N Novolin N	NPH (N)	1 to 3 hours	8 hours	12 to 16 hours
Long-acting	Levemir	Insulin detemir	1 hour	Peakless	20 to 26 hours
	Lantus	Insulin glargine			
Pre-mixed NPH (intermediate-acting) and regular (short-acting)	Humulin 70/30 Novolin 70/30	70% NPH and 30% regular	30 to 60 minutes	Varies	10 to 16 hours
	Humulin 50/50	50% NPH and 50% regular	30 to 60 minutes	Varies	10 to 16 hours
Pre-mixed insulin lispro protamine suspension (intermediate-acting) and insulin lispro (rapid-acting	Humalog Mix 75/25	75% insulin lispro protamine and 25% insulin lispro	10 to 15 minutes	Varies	10 to 16 hours
	Humalog Mix 50/50	50% insulin lispro protamine and 50%	10 to 15 minutes	Varies	10 to 16 hours

Source:
NIH.gov(http://diabetes.niddk.nih.gov/dm/pubs/medicines_ez/insert_C.aspx)

Common Drug Stems
Source NIH.gov
(http://druginfo.nlm.nih.gov/drugportal/jsp/drugportal/DrugNameGenericStems.jsp)

Stem	Drug Class
-adol or -aldol-	Analgesics
-alol	Combined alpha and beta blockers
-arone	Antiarrhythmics
-aril	Antiviral
-teplase	Enzymes; tissue plasminogen activators
-azepam	Antianxiety
-barb or barb-	Barbituric acid derivatives
-cef	Cephlosporins
-coxib	Cyclooxygenase-2 inhibitors
-cort-	Cortisone derivatives
-conazole	Systemic antifungals
-dil-, dil-, or - dil	Vasodilators
-mycin	Antibiotic
nal-	Narcotic agonist/antagonist
-olol	Beta-blockers
-olone	Steroids
-pamil	Coronary vasodilators
-perone	Antianxiety agents
-pezil	Acetylcholinesterase inhibitors
-pidem	Hypnotics/sedative
-prazole	Antiulcer agent
-pressin	Vasoconstrictors
-pril	ACE inhibitors
-sartan	ARBs
-semide	Diuretic
-sporin	Immunosuppressants
-terol	Bronchodilators
-thiazide	Diuretics
-tricin	Antibiotics
-vir, -vir-, vir-	Antiviral

Common Critical Care Drips
Check with you institutional policies prior to starting or titrating ANY drip

Drug	Brand Name	Dose	Use	Other
Nicardipine	Cardene	5-15 mg/hr	decrease BP	Ca Channel Blocker - Do NOT give with nimotop
Norepinephrine	Levophed	5-30 mcg/min	Increase BP	
Fentanyl	Sublimaze	25-200 mcg/hr	Pain Control	
Propofol	Diprivan	20-200 mcg/kg/min	Sedation	SAT RASS
Versed	Midazolam	1-10 mg/hr	Sedation	SAT RASS
Vasopressin	Pitressin	units/min	DI, Sepsis, hypotension	ADH - Titrate to urine output -Cause decreased Urine Specific Gravity
Heparin		units/kr/hr	Anticoagulation	Draw PTT (blue top)
Insulin		units	Decrease BS	
Neosnyphrine	phenylephrine	40-200 mcg/min	Increase BP	
Dexmedetomidine	Precedex	0.1-0.7 mcg/kg/hr	Sedation	SAT RASS

Common Light Sensitive Drugs

Partial list of common medications that are light sensitive. Consult drug guide, pharmacist, and institutional guidelines prior to administering any medication.

Acylovir tab
Adrenaline inj
Aminophylline/Theophylline
Amlodipine + HCTZ
Atropine Sulfate inj
Atenolol tab
Ceftriaxone inj
Dexamethasone inj
Diazepam tab/inj
Digoxin
Fluoxetine tab
Furosemide tab/inj
Losartan potassium tab
Metoprolol tab
Nifedipine cap
Naloxone inj
Proporanolol tab
Rifampin tab
Thyroxin tab

Source:
(http://www.pharmyaring.com/download/doc100122083450.pdf)

Celsius to Fahrenheit Conversion

Celsius	Fahrenheit
36	96.8
36.1	96.98
36.2	97.16
36.4	97.52
36.5	97.7
36.7	98.06
36.8	98.24
36.9	98.42
37	98.6
37.1	98.78
37.2	98.96
37.4	99.32
37.5	99.5
37.6	99.68
37.8	100.04
37.9	100.22
38	100.4
38.1	100.58
38.2	100.76
38.4	101.12
38.5	101.3
38.6	101.48
38.8	101.84
38.9	102.02
39	102.2
39.1	102.38
39.2	102.56
39.4	102.92
39.5	103.1
39.6	103.28
39.8	103.64
39.9	103.82
40	104
40.1	104.18
40.2	104.36
40.4	104.72
40.5	104.9
40.6	105.08
40.8	105.44

40.9	105.62
41	105.8

Nursing Calculations

$$\frac{Ordered}{Have} = Dose$$

$$\frac{Concentration\ \%}{100} X\ Volume = Dosage\ Amount$$

$$\frac{Volume}{Time} = Flow\ Rate$$

$$\frac{Volume(mL)}{Time\ (minutes)}\ x\ Drop\ Factor\ \left(\frac{gtts}{mL}\right) = Flow\ Rate\ (\frac{gtts}{minute})$$

weight in Kg * Dose per Kg = Required Dose

$$\frac{weight\ (kg)}{height(meter)^2} = BMI$$

Nursing Math Conversions

1 teaspoon (t) = 5 ml
1 tablespoon (T) = 3 t = 15 ml
1 oz = 30 ml
1 cup = 8 oz
1 quart = 2 pints
1 pint = 2 cups
1 grain (gr) = 60 mg
1 gram (g) = 1,000 mg
1 kilogram (kg) = 2.2 lbs
1 lb = 16 oz

APGAR Scoring

	0	1	2
Appearance	Blue or pale	Blue at extremities, body pink	No cyanosis, body and extremities pink
Pulse Rate	Absent	<100 bpm	>100 bpm
Reflex Irritability	No response to stimulation	Grimace on suction or stimulation	Flexed arms and legs that resist extension
Activity	None	Some flexion	Flexed arms and legs resist extension
Respiratory Effort	Absent	Weak, irregular, gasping	Strong, lusty cry

Breath Sounds

Wheeze or rhonchi	continuous	high (wheeze) or lower (ronchi)	expiratory or inspiratory	whistling/sibilant, musical	asthma, many others
Stridor	continuous	high	either, mostly inspiratory	whistling/sibilant, musical	epiglottitis, foreign body, laryngeal oedema, croup
Inspiratory gasp	continuous	high	inspiratory	whoop	pertussis (whooping cough)
Crackles (rales)	discontinuous	high or low, nonmusical	inspiratory	cracking/clicking/rattling	pneumonia, congestive heart failure

Maslow Hierarchy of Needs

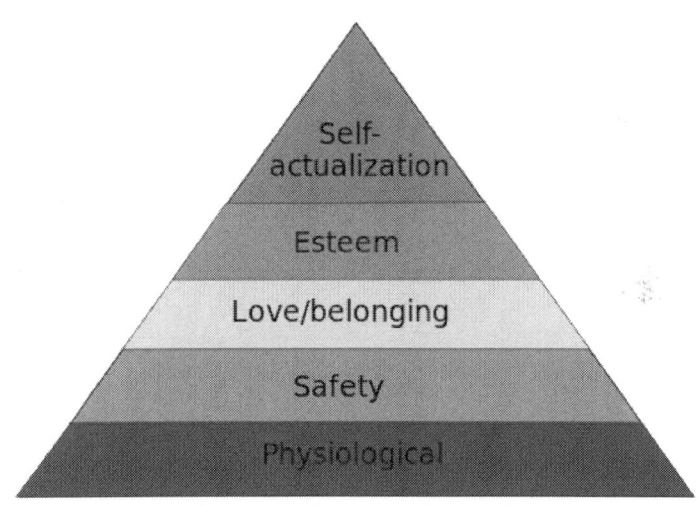

Head to Toe Assessment Checklist

Recommended order for head to toe assessment-not intended to be a complete assessment guide.

- General Assessment
- Body Structure/Mobility
- Behavior
- Health History
- Vital Signs
    - Height Weight
    - Pulse Rate
    - Respirations
    - Temperature
    - Blood Pressure
    - Pain
- Integumentary
    - Inspect: color, moisture, hair, rashes, lesions, pallor, edema
    - Palpate: temperature, turgor, lesions, edema, texture
- Scalp
    - Inspect: shape, symmetry
    - Palpate: tenderness, deformity
- Nails
    - Inspect: shape, color
    - Palpate: capillary refill
- Head
    - Inspect: symmetry, shape, size, uniformity
- Neck
    - Inspect: symmetry, lesions, scars
    - Palpate: tenderness, lymph nodes, thyroid gland, TMJ
- Eyes
    - Inspect: interior and exterior, visual fields, acuity, reflexes
- Ears
    - Inspect: color, shape, symmetry, interior inspection
    - Palpate: tenderness, deformity
- Nose

- - Inspect: shape, symmetry, interior inspection
  - Palpate: frontal sinus, maxillary sinuses
- Mouth and Throat
  - Inspect: exterior and interior
- Thorax and Lungs (anterior and posterior)
  - Inspection: respiration quality, symmetry, deformity, tracheal location
  - Palpation: tenderness, fremitus, chest expansion
  - Percussion: percussive tones, diaphragmatic excursion
  - Auscultation: breath sounds and quality
- Heart and Great Vessels
  - Inspection: jugular venous pulse
  - Palpate: pulses, PMI
  - Auscultate: heart sounds (bell and diaphragm)
- Peripheral Vascular System
  - Inspect: color, edema
  - Palpate: temperature, edema
- Abdomen
  - Inspect: discomfort, uniformity, color, symmetry, scars, hernia, peristalsis, pulsations
  - Auscultate: bowel sounds, bruits
  - Percussion: four quadrants, liver, spleen, renal tenderness
  - Palpation: light to deep, liver, spleen, aorta, rebound tenderness, fluid wave
- Musculoskeletal
  - Inspection: asymmetry, deformity, atrophy
  - Palpation: major joints, tenderness, deformity, range of motion
- Neurological
  - Inspect: mental status (health history), cranial nerves, coordination, movement, senses
  - Palpate: motor strength, muscle tone, reflexes, senses
- Genitourinary
  - Inspect: general appearance, lesions, scars
  - Palpate: breast exam, testicular exam, prostate exam, vaginal exam, Pap smear

- Lymphatic
  - Palpate: assess lymph node locations

Adult Vital Signs

HR: 60-100 bpm
RR: 12-20 rpm
BP: <120/<80 mmHg (heart.org)
Temp: 37°C (98.6°F)

Your Free Gift!
As a way of saying thanks for your purchase, I'm offering a free
PDF download:

"63 Must Know NCLEX® Labs"

With these charts you will be able to take the 63 most important
labs with you anywhere you go!
You can download the 4 page PDF document by going to
NRSNG.com/labs

Made in the USA
Columbia, SC
05 August 2017